Penguin Books

Penguin Nursing

CARE FOR THE ELDERLY

Other titles in this series:

Ear, Nose and Throat Nursing
General Medical Nursing
Ophthalmic Nursing
Orthopaedic Nursing
Principles of Nursing
Surgical Nursing

Jenny Shaw.

Penguin Nursing Revision Notes
Advisory Editor: P. A. Downie

■ Care for the Elderly

Penny A. Hollingham, BA, RGN, SCM, RNT
Tutor, Broadland School of Nursing, Norwich

Penguin Books

PENGUIN BOOKS

Published by the Penguin Group
27 Wrights Lane, London W 8 5 T Z, England
Viking Penguin Inc., 40 West 23rd Street, New York, New York 10010, U S A
Penguin Books Australia Ltd, Ringwood, Victoria, Australia
Penguin Books Canada Ltd, 2801 John Street, Markham, Ontario, Canada L 3 R 1 B 4
Penguin Books (N Z) Ltd, 182–190 Wairau Road, Auckland 10, New Zealand

Penguin Books Ltd, Registered Offices: Harmondsworth, Middlesex, England

First published 1990
10 9 8 7 6 5 4 3 2 1

Copyright © Penguin Books Ltd, 1990
All rights reserved

Made and printed in Great Britain by
Cox and Wyman Ltd, Reading, Berks.
Typeset in 9/10½pt Linotron 202 Galliard by
Rowland Phototypesetting Ltd, Bury St Edmunds, Suffolk

Except in the United States of America, this book is sold subject
to the condition that it shall not, by way of trade or otherwise, be lent,
re-sold, hired out, or otherwise circulated without the
publisher's prior consent in any form of binding or cover other than
that in which it is published and without a similar condition
including this condition being imposed on the subsequent purchaser

Contents

Advisory editor's note

This series of revision aids first saw the light of day in the early 1980s, and the books have been reprinted numerous times, thus indicating that they fulfil a real need. They have now been revised and updated. This particular title, *Care for the Elderly*, has been rewritten, and the emphasis is on a sociological understanding of the elderly and the implications for nursing care which stem from this.

The self-examination questions which have been a most important feature of the series are also set out differently. Because the questions require an essay-type answer it has not been possible to provide factual answers, as in the other titles; instead, outline answers will be found in a complete section at the end of the book. It is suggested that nurses should draft their own answers and then turn to the section to check that all the suggested points have been included.

The convention of referring to the patient as 'he' has been observed in most cases throughout the book; similarly the nurse as 'she'. The reason is one of expediency which allows easier reading. It is not sexist.

In the 1850s Florence Nightingale, discussing how to teach nurses to nurse, wrote in her *Notes on Nursing*: 'I do not pretend to teach her how, I ask her to teach herself, and for this purpose I venture to give her some hints.' Now, some hundred years on, it falls to Penguin Books to offer 'some hints' to the learner nurse of the present day as she prepares for her examinations.

P.D.
Norwich, 1989

1 The aged person in society

Growing old like growing up is part of man's life cycle; it is influenced by a person's experience of life, social and work experience and the ability of the person to adapt to the changes that occur. Old age can be happy or sad and this can affect the people around the older person, the family and social contacts. One in six of the population is over 65, and it is estimated that a third of our lives is spent in retirement.

■ AGEISM

This term applies to the labelling or stereotyping of particular age-groups such as toddlers or teenagers. In recent years the elderly have been labelled *en masse*, e.g. geriatrics, as a group; this denies them individuality and expects them to conform to an 'old' stereotype. The discrimination against elderly people just because they are old is described by Gray and Wilcock (1981) 'ageism is as reprehensible as racism or sexism and it can be as damaging and demeaning to individuals.' It is important for the nurse to recognize people's concepts of old age, to study the writings about the old, and to recognize the truth from the subjective opinion of others who may refer to the elderly in derogatory terms. Those terms are often 'gerries', 'grannies', 'oldies', 'grandads', 'geriatrics'. Most older people resent being referred to as 'geriatric' which has senile implications to the lay public. Our Western society frequently underestimates the value of our older people. The media are quick to record an older person's age if they do something that is at all unusual or untypical, which would not be recorded for someone younger. In many Eastern societies the old person is venerated and consulted as a wise member of the community. The Jewish communities in the kibbutz don't have any retirement ages; all the families regardless of age help one another as a community no matter how small the contribution. In this way the older member of the community retains self-esteem and worth.

Many famous politicians have produced their best speeches in their 80s and 90s like Churchill and Lord Stockton. Many famous artists have painted some of their finest pictures and works of art in later life. Throughout the years, men and women have achieved greatness in their later years. Not many of us will be a Picasso, Haydn or Shaw, but there are many positive aspects to old age. It would be good to think that each individual can have time in retirement to develop potential for living, whether to achieve greatness or just to enjoy hobbies or develop skills or interests. It is possible that a person will be more creative in old age than when they were younger.

Our society depends on its capitalist economy and the acquisition of wealth, so it is understandable that the workforce needs to be young and fit; therefore older people may be regarded as an economic burden. The working life ends in retirement with the receipt of the old age pension at 65 for men and 60 for women, the exception being a few professionals such as doctors, judges, politicians and the self-employed.

It is a fallacy to think that all older people will be a burden to the state; the majority of older people are self-sufficient, will be prepared for old age, and live in their own homes.

■ THE PRIVILEGED AND UNDER-PRIVILEGED

Today more than ever before people need to prepare financially for retirement; if a person has been in a low-paid job, or unemployed, then saving is not possible. Living on just an old age pension will reduce standards of living and cause hardship and real poverty.

There is no doubt that money can bring the material things of life, access to private medicine, better food, long holidays. Today the active young elderly or 'woopies' (well-off older people of 60–69 years), are able to spend their money freely to enjoy life to the limit.

A considerable number of people undertake a part-time job when they retire, to bring in an extra income. The young elderly, or 'young old' are classed as 65–75 and the 'old old' 75–85+ (Isaacs et al, 1972). The young elderly frequently fulfil an active social role within society, helping other members of the family, such as minding the grandchildren while the daughter goes out to work. Voluntary work is frequently undertaken, such as meals on wheels, WRVS work or manning the hospital car service. Charity organizations depend on older people for manpower, so do local and parish councils. This fills the gaps in society which cannot be filled by younger working men and women. ·

■ DEMOGRAPHIC CHANGES

By the year 2000 it is estimated that there will be a decrease in the number of people between the ages of 65–70, and an increase in the number of people over 80. This has an implication for the planning of care in the twenty-first century. Due to the present low birth rate the number of young adults available to care for the elderly is decreasing. Bosanquet (1978) states 'that it is usually held that a person over 75 years uses health and social services eight times more than the normal equivalent adult!'

■ **The reason for the demographic changes**

Over the last hundred years Britain like other Western industrialized societies has reduced its birth rate, and lowered its infant mortality rate. People are not only surviving to old age but living to a much greater age. The life expectancy of a girl surviving to old age is still greater than that for a boy, and several suggestions have been made for this. It is thought that boys are more daring and take more risks, and that they undertake more hazardous work in mines and on oil rigs. They are also more likely to suffer military mortality. In the past men have drunk and smoked more than women and suffered from more occupational diseases. It has been found that the proportion of women to men rises with age, and the men that do survive are usually physically in better condition than women.

■ **The reason why men and women are living longer**

This has been brought about initially by improved environmental factors such as better housing, safe water and disposal of waste and refuse, and improved food hygiene. Education and health knowledge, improved standards of living and social changes influencing parents in planning families, improved working conditions and the prevention of accidents have all helped towards better health. Immunization programmes have reduced the number of the killer infectious diseases, such as diphtheria, measles, polio, whooping cough, etc. Scientific, medical, technical and nursing knowledge have helped to reduce disease and enabled treatment for many of the incurable diseases of the past. For example, an epidural anaesthetic can now be given instead of a general anaesthetic for an elderly person requiring a hip replacement or the repair of a fractured femur. The postoperative complications are reduced, with less risk of chest infections and hypostatic pneumonia.

■ **The distribution patterns of the elderly in Britain**

In Britain the retirement migration has been predominantly to the coastal resorts. The most popular resorts have been in East Anglia, the South-West, the outer parts of the South-East region, North Wales, Lancashire and the Yorkshire coast. About 10 per cent of the population move every year in Britain and the elderly form a small part of this migration from the large cities to rural and coastal regions. There are many problems that occur when elderly couples move to country cottages or bungalows by the sea, that look so attractive during the summer. Moving house and retirement are considered stressful life events; these in themselves can contribute to the onset of illness. The older a couple the more difficult it is for them to become accepted into a new neighbourhood and to obtain help in times of illness. Inevitably when one or other partner dies, health and social problems occur. This need will be met by the caring services, but resources are badly stretched. An example of this can be seen in the Norwich Health District; at the census date 1985, 15 per cent of the population of England and Wales was over 65; East Anglia was 16 per cent and Norwich Health District 18 per cent, with some areas on the North Norfolk coast reaching 23 per cent (Sheringham and Cromer). MacDonald (1988) states that the resorts along England's South Coast are being turned into mass retirement homes. Seaton in South Devon – 'Elderly outnumber the young by two to one!'

■ Social implications of these demographic changes

The size of the average family has decreased, with fewer children to care for parents. There are fewer unmarried daughters to stay at home than there were in the past. Today the daughter works, and the proportion of women who marry has grown steadily. Frequently sons and daughters move away from their parents to obtain work and settle down some distance away with their own families and friends, so that the elderly parents are left on their own. Frequently the husband dies first. If he is the only car driver in a rural area the wife cannot get out and about. Despite this, families still remain the main care support, but with the burden falling on one member, usually a daughter, rather than being shared.

■ Loneliness and isolation

These problems can occur if there are no friends or family near by, particularly if the elderly person is house-bound as a result of a physical disability such as arthritis. Loneliness and isolation can be as big a problem to the elderly person marooned in a house or flat in an inner city as that of an elderly person in a bungalow by the sea. The bungalow by the sea is not so attractive in the winter months when the wind howls round and the elderly person is alone and no one calls.

■ REFERENCES

Bosanquet, N. (1978). *A Future for Old Age. Towards a New Society*, p. 7. Temple Smith, London.

Gray, M. and Wilcock, G. (1981). *Our Elders*, p. 33. Oxford University Press, Oxford.

Isaacs, B., Livingstone, M. and Neville, Y. (1972). *Survival of the Unfittest*, p. 17. Routledge, London.

MacDonald, E. (1988). GPs prescribed seaside ban on pensioners. *The Observer*, 25 October.

■ SELF-EXAMINATION QUESTIONS

1 Why are people living longer, and what has brought about the changes?
2 Do you think that the number of very old people in the community is putting a greater strain on financial resources? How should this problem be overcome?
3 Do you think loneliness and isolation can be a problem to older people? How can this be prevented?

2 The ageing process and nursing implications

■ THE AGEING PROCESS

There are many theories about how and why ageing occurs and what triggers the ageing process, which will eventually end in death. Most people would agree that there are some hereditary links. If a person comes from a family whose parents and grandparents live to a great age, then it is highly probable that he will too. The reason why some families live longer than others may be due to factors that influence the ageing process and the speed at which ageing occurs.

■ The effects of the physical environment and ageing

Harsh environmental conditions that are caused by chemicals or radiation can have an adverse effect on the cellular structure of the body. Micro-organisms and parasites can also have adverse effects. This is apparent in countries where water and food are infected as a result of poor hygiene and polluted water.

■ Socio-economic factors

Poor living, housing and working conditions, unemployment and poverty can lower standards of living which in turn predispose towards ill-health. Chronic illnesses may well develop which may speed up the ageing process. Bosanquet (1978a) points out that there are important differences between social classes in health standards. Research has been undertaken by the organization Age Concern into the health and fitness of groups of elderly people in terms of their ability to carry out certain activities. This included housework, walking and climbing stairs. The survey suggested that in the different social strata 35 per cent of skilled people in socio-economic groups 1, 2, 3 were fit, but only 19 per cent unskilled and semi-skilled people in socio-economic groups 4, 5 were fit.

■ Personal lifestyle

The care and abuse of the body over the years will affect health. Many of the diseases that commonly occur in old age are not the result of the ageing process but the consequence of having lived for a long time in a certain style. Smoking 40 cigarettes a day over the age of 30–40 will cause respiratory disease, rather than ageing lung tissue. Poor diet and lack of exercise or too much alcohol may all cause ill-health and can shorten life. Any health problems that become chronic will continue into old age. There are *no* illnesses which are found only in old age; arthritis or Alzheimer's disease do occur earlier in life as can diabetes and a stroke. They are, however, more common after 60. Grouping elderly people in sheltered complexes can create an artificial community and give rise to social deprivation.

■ Theories of ageing

These can be divided into psychological and biological theories:

□ *Psychological Theories*
The exchange theory is based on the assumption that interactions between people exist and grow because of the stimulus from this interaction. As a person grows old there is less social interaction and he frequently becomes more isolated and dependent on others.

Role Theory: This suggests loss of social roles, particularly the work role for men, reducing self-esteem and loss of function; there is difficulty in establishing new roles. This can occur with career women.

Disengagement Theory: This suggests that as people grow older there is a disengagement from their role as workers. The older person withdraws from society and its roles: the younger people take over power and control.

The Activity Theory: This suggests that the older person is the same as the middle-aged apart from physical change. Those who stay active and lead a fulfilling life will achieve a satisfying ageing process.

□ *The Biological Theories*
The human body is made up of cells which are constantly dividing and being replaced, and in order for the body to survive this process has to function. Any nutritional deficiency, such as the reduction of oxygen or nutrients, will affect cellular function.

Waste Product Accumulation Theory: The accumulation of waste chemicals from the breakdown of intracellular membranes causes death of cells.

Auto-immune Theory: The immune response to disease is less when a person is old. It has also been found that the ageing body produces antibodies, called auto-antibodies, against healthy tissue.

Programmed Ageing Theory: This may be called the biological clock theory.

It is based on the theory that the body is genetically programmed in the genes which influence cell function, development, maturation and ageing. Several theories have centred on an overall time clock in the brain.

These are some of the more common theories about ageing and there still needs to be further research on this subject. The process of ageing is accelerated if the older person has to contend with a chronic health condition such as rheumatoid arthritis, physical deformity, congenital defects or mental illness.

■ PHYSIOLOGICAL CHANGES WITH THEIR NURSING IMPLICATIONS

Ageing varies with each individual, and as already mentioned there are many factors that influence this process. When ageing occurs it will affect all the cells of the body and will gradually reduce the number and size of the cells. The body fat atrophies with very advanced age giving the body a bony appearance. Intracellular fluid decreases and so does total body fluid.

1   To summarize the nursing implications relating to physiology of ageing

Physiological changes	Nursing implications
Outward body appearance	
Skin	
(a) The first change that an older person notices is in the skin. It becomes drier; wrinkles and sagging occur. This is partially due to the loss of subcutaneous fat, and inelasticity of muscles and skin	Because the skin is more delicate and drier it is often more appropriate to use moisturizers, rather than talcum powder, when caring for an older person's hygiene needs
(b) The skin is more fragile and bruises easily. There are spotty pigmentations in areas exposed to the sun, e.g. back of the hands and arms	If knocked the skin can break. There is a danger of pressure sores if the older person is confined to bed or chair (Goldstone and Goldstone, 1982; Waterlow, 1985)
(c) Reduced blood supply to the skin and subcutaneous tissue; decrease in immune system, in the antibody and neutrophil production and mitotic growth of epithelial cells. Slow response to haemostatic mechanisms of the body	Wounds heal more slowly. If a pressure sore develops, more difficult to heal

Physiological changes	Nursing implications
(d) Atrophy of the sweat glands and a decrease in the blood supply	Protection of the skin; suitable clothing according to weather
(e) The skin cannot regulate the external temperature so effectively. This can be due to the loss of subcutaneous fat which acts as an insulator	Avoidance of hypothermia. Avoidance of chilling due to undue exposure. May need warmer environment and clothes than younger people

Nails

Grow more slowly and are thick and irregular particularly toenails	It may be necessary to assist the older person to cut nails or arrange for a chiropodist to visit

Hair

Becomes thinner and greyer. Some women grow more facial hair due to hormone imbalance	Removal of facial hair to improve body image

Body movement

The muscle power of an older person gradually becomes less over the years. There is less strength and tone due to loss of muscle mass; Cormack (1985) quotes a study that shows a decline in the hand-grip power of an older person:	Important to encourage movement of all muscles with regular exercise not only to prevent muscle weakness and loss of function but also to encourage strength, tone and stamina
Hand grip pressure: 35-yr-old – 45kg 85-yr-old – 20–25kg In both sexes the grip of the dominant hand was greater	The grip of a very old person is sometimes feeble – special fittings may be needed, e.g. to turn a tap or hold a toothbrush
As age increases all the major muscles of the body become weaker – due to the decrease in muscle fibres. Muscles in arms and legs reduced in size and flabby	If a patient is chair- or bed-bound it is important to prevent muscle wasting by encouraging bed exercises
Slower reaction time	Older people may be unable to walk as fast, cross a road, or get out of an emergency situation

Joints and bones

Elderly people tend to get a characteristic curve of the spine – *kyphosis*. The head and neck are bent forward when a person stands erect. This is due to a decrease in elasticity, and calcification of ligaments, shrinkage and sclerosis of tendons and changes in the vertebral column with flattening of the intervertebral discs. Body height may decrease by 1–4 inches from young adulthood. Loss of muscle and bone mass	Encourage regular exercise to prevent loss of muscle and bone mass Exercise helps to maintain a more erect posture Support with a stick or walking aid may be necessary Ensure a safe environment for the older person. A fall may result in a fracture

Physiological changes	Nursing implications

Common conditions in older people

(a) *Osteoporosis* is more common in women than men. Caused by a leaching of calcium from the bone matrix; bones become lighter and brittle. Women may have a reduction of oestrogen causing this condition – a fall may result in a fracture

Ensure a safe environment as a fall may result in a fracture

(b) *Osteomalacia* causes brittle bones, fractures, general aches and pains and muscle weakness. It is caused by lack of calcium, due to lack of vitamin D

To prevent both these conditions occurring it is necessary to ensure a good nutritious diet for the older person. Calcium supplement if necessary; and foods containing vitamin D

Joints

The articulating surfaces of the joints may change with the 'wear and tear' over the years. Movement may be more difficult and painful

Physiotherapy for maintaining movement
Treatment of pain for painful joints
Awareness by nursing and medical staff of mobility problems

The heart and circulation

The heart of a healthy individual may be unaffected by ageing. The size may be reduced due to the reduction of physical activity – this in turn results in reduction of cardiac output. Valves may become rigid. There is a longer interval between contractions due to weakened contractile strength of the muscles

Regular exercise according to the age and fitness of the older person to ensure cardiac function. A very old person needs more time for the heart rate to return to normal after exercise

Physical changes in old age

Blood pressure increases in both sexes, with the systolic increasing more than the diastolic due to an increase of peripheral resistance. Arteriosclerosis of the vessels increases the peripheral resistance. The heart therefore has to pump harder against this increased resistance.
Atherosclerosis may be present in some vessels

It is normal to record a slightly higher blood pressure for an older person

Breathing

The ageing lung tissue loses its elasticity, the number of alveoli are reduced and increased in size. This means the older person does not breathe as efficiently as a younger person. The vital capacity of the lungs are reduced; an older person takes smaller breaths

If an older person has to stay in bed, breathing exercises to prevent the development of a chest infection particularly *hypostatic pneumonia* should be taught by the physiotherapist. If an older person is ill visitors with colds should be discouraged

Physiological changes	Nursing implications
Kyphosis reduces the movement of the rib cage. This makes the older person more susceptible to infection. There is less ventilation at the base of the lungs and more at the apex	If an older person requires an anaesthetic this can cause postoperative problems

Eating

The older person's gums recede with age; some teeth may be lost	Good oral hygiene and regular dental checks. The prevention of gum disease and cavities. Ensure well-fitting dentures so that food can be chewed and enjoyed. Speaking will be easier if dentures are worn
Taste and smell	
These senses deteriorate with age; taste buds decrease; the older person will season food to make it taste	Important to provide tasty food, to tempt the appetite
Volume of saliva is reduced	
Salivary amylase is reduced which will affect starch digestion	This may result in chewing difficulties; swallowing may not be so easy if food is dry. Starchy food may cause indigestion
The digestion of food	
There is decreased peristaltic movement in the stomach and intestine and less gastric secretion. The emptying of the lower oesophageal sphincter is slower. Slower absorption of substances through the stomach and intestines as a result of reduced blood flow in the intestinal area and a reduction in digestive enzymes	Older people like smaller regular meals that are attractive and tempting. Good nutritional diet rich in iron, vitamins and poor absorption can result in anaemia and deficiency diseases
Constipation is a common problem, due to decreased muscle tone of the large intestine. If the rectal sphincter is over-relaxed faecal incontinence may occur	Prevent constipation with increased fluid intake in hot weather and a high fibre diet. The nurse should ensure privacy for the patient to have his/her bowels open regularly

Special senses

Hearing	
High frequency tones may not be heard so easily. There may be some loss of hearing due to a deterioration in the hearing mechanism, such as changes in the cochlea and absence of the hearing cells in the organ of Corti. The deafness could be just due to wax	Early recognition and referral to an ENT department. If no treatment is considered a hearing aid can be given to overcome deafness. Isolation and confusion can be caused if speech cannot be understood

Physiological changes	Nursing implications
Balance	
There may be altered perception of a person's position which causes older people to sway	Nurse should be aware of any disturbance of balance; rails round toilets and baths, walking aids may be needed
Sight	
Sight usually deteriorates as a person gets older.	Regular sight testing and the provision of suitable spectacles.
Presbyopia – the decreased ability of the eyes to accommodate for close and distant vision. Pupil size is smaller; less light reaches the retina; papillary constriction and dilation is less efficient. The older person's eyes cannot adapt to dim light and darkness. Less discriminating colour recognition	The older person needs more light by which to see
Conditions affecting the eye	
Cataracts occur in 35% of the elderly. Some older people may develop *macular degeneration* which results in peripheral vision only	Early recognition and treatment of any sight problems
Re-absorption of the intra-ocular fluid is less efficient and may lead to eventual breakdown of absorption process, which creates potential for *glaucoma*	Instillation of eyedrops may be necessary
The lubrication and cleansing action of the lacrimal secretions is less. Eyes may feel dry and irritable	Eyes may need to be bathed more frequently
Many people over 65 develop a white line that encircles or partially encircles periphery of the iris known as *arcus senilis*	
Feeling	
The touch receptors are less efficient. An older person is less able to make fine movements. This may be frustrating to some people if they have less sensitivity to touch and to heat and cold	The very old person may need help in sewing on buttons or holding fine objects

The brain

There is a loss in the total number of brain cells and their fibres with advanced age.
Loss of brain weight 20–25% from maturity to 90.
There may be arteriosclerotic changes which affect the cerebral arterial system.

Nurses need to be aware of the worry patients have of losing their memory, or the thought that they may be considered senile. Many older people are capable of higher intellectual reasoning and thought if given *time* and can be just as accurate as a young

Physiological changes	Nursing implications
Short-term memory deteriorates; older people usually remember what they did in their youth but cannot always remember immediate behaviour, e.g. whether they have put the kettle on.	person. Aids may be required to remind the older person about the present time or immediate needs
Motor movements slow down, reaction time reduced	Give the older person time to respond. Walking will be slower; – need longer time to cross a busy road

Sleeping

Sleep patterns may change if the older person is less active during the day, and has short sleeps in daylight hours. Some elderly people like going early to bed then rise early	Help the older person have a healthy sleep pattern of their choice. Increase activity in the day, avoid anxiety; relaxation exercises or massage to improve relaxation

Sexuality

In women the walls of the vagina become drier. *Vaginitis* is common. Reproductive activity is not lost in older men but spermatozoa decrease. Sexual performance may decline with years. Sexual enjoyment and activity continue into old age	Older people should be encouraged to take a healthy normal view of sex, if they so wish

Production of urine and bladder function

The renal blood flow to the kidneys is reduced, as a result of decreased cardiac output. This in turn reduces the filtration rate in the kidneys	Older people frequently need to pass urine during the night – may get up once or twice. The nurse should ensure there is a light and access to a lavatory, commode or urinal within reach
Men may get prostate enlargement. 75% of men over 55 have problems	
Some women may get urgency or stress incontinence due to poor pelvic muscle floor support	Women with stress incontinence and urgency may benefit from pelvic floor exercises. If necessary referral may be made to a gynaecologist for treatment

Older person's response to pain

There is a diminished pain response in the elderly. People over 60 are said to have a higher pain tolerance than those under 60. This reduced pain response in older people can mask serious conditions such as those of the abdomen and heart	Careful assessment of the older person to ascertain the severity and position of the pain. Gentle handling and reassurance of the older person. Treatment according to the medical prescription

■ THE ADJUSTMENT OF AN OLDER PERSON TO THE PROCESS OF GROWING OLD

Ageing is a gradual process and comes upon us all in an insidious way. Throughout life a person is constantly adapting to change, from childhood to adulthood, to worker and possibly parenthood. As age progresses one role is relinquished for another. People learn to handle the best ways to adapt to their changes. In order to prepare for the final change from the world of work to retirement it is useful if the older person obtains advice. This will improve his/her knowledge to change attitudes and develop skills to enjoy retirement to the fullest. Many firms, local health and education authorities and industrial organizations run pre-retirement courses. Figure 1 shows a framework of the aims of a course.

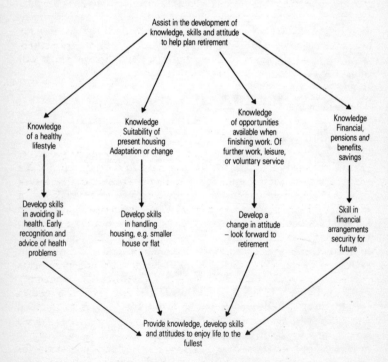

Fig. 1 Pre-retirement preparation

■ RETIREMENT

In the past, retirement has been to many people a social disaster: they have been unprepared for the world of leisure, on the 'scrap heap'. Today, with adequate preparation a pensioner should look forward to retirement, know his rights, be very much fitter to enjoy life, or to carry on part-time work. Problems inevitably occur if there is chronic physical or mental ill-health, if there has been unemployment and no means to save anything towards retirement, if the housing is badly maintained or there is over-crowding. Bosanquet (1978b) wrote 'To retire is for many people to step on a time machine and to move backwards in terms of living standards.' He went on to describe how many people who are used to independence choose to spend their money – 'The poor elderly on a reduced pension spend most of their money on the three basic necessities; food, housing and heat.' The greatest deprivation felt by the elderly is to be unable to take a holiday. Again, according to Bosanquet (1978c) the Age Concern survey shows that 42 per cent of a sample of old people had not had a holiday for two years, including weekends. In order for older people to enjoy retire-ment, maintain standards of living and a suitable lifestyle which will enhance life, it is necessary to have enough money.

■ CONCLUSION

Preparation for old age is important for people from all socio-economic groups, not only to prepare for the material things of life, but for the changes that will affect status and self-esteem as a pensioner. The loss of companionship in the workplace can cause loneliness for many people, if there is nothing to fill their place of work. Good health enables a person to live life to the fullest. In order to keep fit in old age it is necessary to continue a healthy lifestyle, to have a balanced, healthy and nutritious diet, to avoid excesses in life such as too much alcohol and smoking, and to exercise to maintain body function and mobility. Such organizations as 'Extend' (exercises for the elderly) are ideal for the over 60s. Swimming, cycling, walking, golf and many other activities that a person is used to enjoying should be encouraged as long as possible. Many clubs and local authorities have reduced fees for pensioners. Further education courses provide intellectual and social companionship.

There are political problems to be resolved in order to provide health for all by the year 2000, as proposed by the World Health Organization for Europe. Housing for the elderly is still insufficient and lacking in many rural and urban areas. Financial benefits for the elderly are still inadequate for many people, who have no savings.

It is the unfit 'old old' 75+ who are the most vulnerable.

■ REFERENCES

Bosanquet, N. (1978a). *A Future for Old Age. Towards a New Society*, p. 23. Temple Smith, London.

Bosanquet, N. (1978b). *A Future for Old Age. Towards a New Society*, p. 45. Temple Smith, London.

Bosanquet, N. (1978c). *A Future for Old Age. Towards a New Society*, p. 47. Temple Smith, London.

Cormack, D. (ed.) (1985). *Geriatric Nursing. A Conceptual Approach*, p. 59. Blackwell Scientific Publications Limited, Oxford.

Goldstone, L. A. and Goldstone, J. (1982). The Norton score: an early warning of pressure. *Journal of Advanced Nursing*, 7, 419–20.

Waterlow, J. (1985). A risk assessment card. *Nursing Times*, **81**, 48, 49–55.

■ SELF-EXAMINATION QUESTIONS

1 Name some of the theories of ageing.

2 What is the Norton pressure sore at-risk calculator and why should it be used?

3 How does the Waterlow at-risk calculator differ from the Norton at-risk calculator?

4 Why are older people more likely to develop hypothermia? How can it be prevented?

5 Why should an older person be more at risk from developing hypostatic pneumonia?

6 For what reasons would you recommend pre-retirement preparation for older people?

7 What precautions should be taken to ensure that older people do not have an accident while in hospital?

3 A holistic approach to care

To meet all an individual's needs it is essential to look at the whole person, not just a part (Fig. 2). This is particularly important when dealing with the health and well-being of older people. One should not look at him/her in isolation from the environment. It is necessary to look at the person's ability to cope at home, a person's previous knowledge, occupation and his social needs and aspirations in order to understand the older person better. It may be necessary to arrange for financial assistance if health is affected by poverty or hardship, for example the house may be inadequately heated, and the older person is admitted to hospital with hypothermia. In this case the environmental needs are not being met; maybe this is because of lack of money which causes a physiological problem.

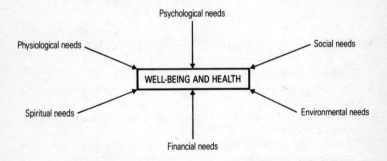

Fig. 2 The areas of need that should be assessed

One of the main reasons for the elderly to seek advice and help from a doctor or nurse is when they have an illness causing a physiological or psychological problem. This could be caused because the other health needs have not been met. On the other hand the illness can affect other areas of need.

Maslow (1954) published his theory of motivation which showed how an individual's needs (to have health and well-being) are a complex interaction between the environment and activity (Fig. 3). Maslow proposed that the needs form a hierarchical pyramid: those at the base of the pyramid are the physiological needs, such as food, water, air, shelter, the elimination of waste and the relief of pain, which are essential for survival; the higher levels of needs are related to meeting an individual's psycho-social needs to give a person some quality of life.

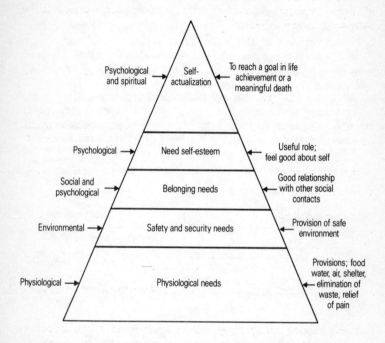

Fig. 3 Hierarchy of human needs, based on Maslow (1954)

Meeting the needs of older people to prevent health problems occurring and to promote independence whenever possible can sometimes be a complicated process. If he is lonely and depressed, dealing with the basic needs of life can be neglected; he may fail to eat properly and become ill, and a cycle of events occurs which may require nursing, medical and social intervention. Man relates to his environment by interacting through the various senses with those around. For example, if an older person is not caring for himself and smells, people will avoid him and isolation and loneliness will occur, he may feel neglected and unwanted and the situation is aggravated.

■ EATING AND DRINKING

There are several factors that need to be considered if an older person is caring for himself to ensure that he is receiving adequate food, that is both nutritious and suitable for his age and cultural needs. Problems arise if he is ill. Figure 4 shows some of the factors needed for a person to be independent and feed himself.

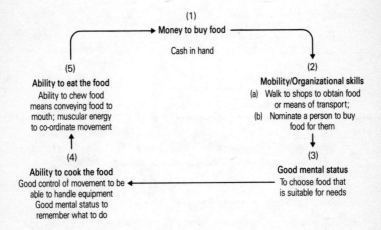

Fig. 4 Factors relating to nutrition, independence and feeding

Figure 4 shows that any break in the chain can result in the older person requiring some help to remain independent. It can be appreciated that insufficient money will lead to a poor diet. For example, when oranges and other fruit are expensive in the winter, the elderly do not buy them, but spend money on fuel to keep warm. As a result they are frequently short of vitamin C in the diet. If an older person has walking difficulties he may be unable to get to a large supermarket where food is cheaper and the variety of goods greater. In order to remain independent he will go to the corner shop, or rely on others to shop for him. Less commonly, poor, short-term memory can affect the choice of food and inability to manage to cook, for example forgetting to turn off the gas, leaving food to burn. If there are any muscular or skeletal problems, cooking may be difficult. Finally, eating the food that is prepared can only be done if a person can cut up the food, which requires manipulation of a knife and fork and this requires muscular energy and co-ordination of movement. The chewing of food requires teeth or well-fitting dentures. In order for him to be independent these factors need to be taken into consideration. If there is any likelihood of a person having difficulties in managing to care for himself, a home assessment is indicated.

■ THE NEED TO MOVE ABOUT

■ Difficulty with mobility

The inability to move about freely where and when one chooses is a major cause of dependence in elderly people. Inability to move from a chair, to go to bed without help or to walk unaided to the toilet may be the first step in a chain of circumstances which can lead to a person being dependent on others.

The pathological problems due to illness, such as a stroke or arthritic disease, or those caused by trauma can affect an older person's mobility and degree of independence. Other diseases causing blindness, deafness and respiratory problems can all reduce his activity. The frustration that he feels about the inability to do what he would normally be able to do can lead to depression.

■ Financial poverty

Someone on a basic pension may be unable to afford to get out and about. This will limit social mobility and can be seen in many rural areas where there is no public transport. If a person cannot afford private transport he can be completely isolated, which may cause not only loss of social contacts but also real problems in buying food and clothing. Some communities in rural areas have overcome this problem. For example, in the Highlands and Islands arrangements are made for the post bus to pick up passengers and take them to local towns. Local tradespeople provide mobile shops, and the mobile library can create a community service providing a meeting place for local people.

■ Bowel function

Because the normal physiological process of digestion is slower in the elderly they are more prone to constipation. This is aggravated if the diet does not contain sufficient fibre, from eating fresh fruit and vegetables and whole cereals. It is also likely that older people do not exercise as regularly. If they are admitted to hospital for treatment the whole daily routine is upset and constipation is a frequent problem.

Faecal incontinence: This is extremely distressing and the most common cause is that of constipation. When there are impacted faeces in the bowel, some of the faeces become liquid as a result of bacterial action, and run down the side of the mass and through the anus.

Nursing needs of the patient require the relief of the constipation and regular toileting to acquire bowel function. Particular care should be taken in skin hygiene to prevent damage to the skin and pressure sores occurring. Regular exercises such as a daily walk should be encouraged.

■ The need for urinary continence

Acquiring the habit of passing urine is a basic skill and socially desirable in order for a person to lead a full independent life. A survey carried out by Thomas et al (1980) reported that 11.6 per cent of women and 6.9 per cent of men over the age of 65 suffered from urinary incontinence.

The loss of dignity and self-esteem, caused by wetting clothes, or the bed or chair, can have disastrous effects on the older person. It is often covered up by him and his relatives, as something 'one doesn't talk about'. Isaacs et al (1972) when discussing incontinence in the elderly at home, said; 'This symptom is the ultimate degradation of old age, causing misery in the patient, a burden of labour to the relatives and a sense of despair to many in the medical and nursing profession'.

Incontinence is more common in older people and its incidence is not affected by marital or family status, housing or social class. The cause of incontinence requires careful assessment by the nurse and the doctor (Table 2). The intelligent use of incontinence aids can cut down the problem of soiling personal clothes and bedding. Nursing intervention and management of the problem can help to improve bladder function, to enable the patient to lead an independent life.

■ THE NEED FOR REST AND SLEEP

Sleep is an extension of rest and both are necessary for survival. Short periods of rest are essential for most old people during the day and are particularly necessary to relieve both psychological and muscular tension. The older a person becomes the more frequently they need short rest periods.

Older people may experience difficulty in going to sleep. This is aggravated if they are worried by something that has occurred during the day. The sleep patterns of the elderly are usually more fragmented than those of the young. There is no doubt that some older people do have disturbed nights and they may lie awake for long periods. This may be due

2 Assessment of urinary incontinence

Causes	Nursing intervention
Environmental	
The older person cannot reach the toilet in time, e.g. walking difficulties	Use of commode/urinal – within reach
	Supply walking aids, assist mobility
Lack of privacy	Ensure privacy
Physiological	
Urinary tract infections	Education of elderly patient to drink more
	Report foul smelling urine
	Blood or pus in the urine
	Frequency of urination
Prostate problems	Report dribbling and frequency and quantity of urine passed
Faecal impaction	Treat any constipation and discomfort
Drug medication	
Toxic confusion due to over-medication, example; diuretics, antidepressants	Report any abnormal behaviour following drug administration
Psychological	
Apathy, depression, anxiety	Report abnormal behaviour, encourage habit training, give encouragement to promote continence

Biggest problem with incontinence is the lack of education, knowledge and awareness by the patient and his relatives and carers.

to leg cramps, nocturnal micturition, or worry. Low-grade depression can be a cause of insomnia.

Nurses should be aware of any disturbance in an older person's sleep pattern, and try and adjust the nursing care to fit into the patient's wishes. For example, being prepared to settle a patient for the night at 9 pm, instead of 11 pm, if this is usual for the patient, who may then be used to getting up at 5 am. A nurse should be able to assess an older person's needs and to provide conditions that are conducive for sleep. Help may be needed to relax the older person at bedtime, by giving him a suitable bedtime drink, repositioning pillows, or blankets, or relieving pain. Soft music from earphones from a bedside radio may lull him to sleep and are better than the use of hypnotics. Sometimes a tot of 'what they fancy' will help them sleep, such as a measure of whisky and water.

■ THE NEED FOR SUITABLE ACCOMMODATION

Most older people will live and die in their own homes and will remain independent as long as they can. Some will remain at home with support from their family and friends. Others need help from the community nursing service, home helps, meals-on-wheels and voluntary and statutory organizations available through the social services department. Whenever possible the older person should be allowed to choose; it has been found that people with the most disabling conditions can remain happy in their own homes no matter how unsuitable they might be considered by outsiders.

Living with relatives: Ideally the older person (or couple) should have a separate room, an annexe or flat, so that privacy and independence may be kept, while sharing meals and having social contacts. Living in crowded accommodation with different generations of a family can bring about problems and lead to friction and arguments.

Sheltered housing: This may be provided by housing departments of local authorities or through private housing schemes such as Anchor Housing associations. Sheltered housing is specifically designed for the elderly and usually consists of flats or bungalows grouped together with a resident warden on site; emergency bells are installed to obtain help. Problems can occur when the elderly are physically and mentally dependent on others for their care – this can result in their being transferred to continuing care, or into residential care thus losing their sheltered flat, or bungalow.

Residential care: Under Part 3 of the National Assistance Act 1948, local authorities are required to provide residential accommodation for people who are unable to care for themselves. This is usually as a result of age or illness. Recently (1988), because of the demand for this type of care more and more private homes have come into being and are registered with the local authority. Many social services departments now pay to send older people to these homes. In addition, there is an increasing problem of accommodating the mentally ill in residential care, as the policy of closing psychiatric hospitals and returning the mentally ill to the community is gradually implemented.

Hospital provision: If an older person has an acute surgical problem he will be admitted to a general hospital for treatment without delay: if he is over 65 and has a medical problem, then treatment may be given in a medical ward of a district general hospital, or a geriatric unit, depending on the local admission procedures, e.g. the age of the patient or the necessity for rehabilitation in a specialized unit for the elderly.

Acute geriatric unit: Such a unit can provide a total approach to patient care. A careful assessment of needs is made and with the help of a multidisciplinary team the patient's problems can be identified; goals can be set and care given to promote health and independence or improved health status.

A psycho-geriatric unit for the elderly: Such a unit admits patients with some psychological disturbance, or disturbance of mental function, that prevents them from living an independent life. Patients are referred in the same way as those referred to a general hospital. A careful assessment of the cause of the illness to exclude a physiological or drug-related cause is made on admission.

National Health Service nursing homes: Small units run by health authorities which are able to provide a holistic type of care for the elderly. The aim is for these units to replace long-stay units.

Day hospitals: These bridge the gap for a patient who may need a certain amount of nursing care and rehabilitation. Patients attend once, twice or three times a week, according to their need.

Social services day centres: These provide respite care for old people. Activities include social and recreational as well as, sometimes, bathing facilities.

Continuing care units for the elderly: Such units are provided for those people with a physical or mental disability who cannot be cared for at home and require continuing nursing care. This type of unit sets out to provide as normal an environment as possible to nurse the elderly infirm.

■ THE NEED TO PROVIDE A SAFE ENVIRONMENT

Research has shown that the majority of falls occur indoors. Despite the utmost care to prevent falls, they will occur. Certain steps can be taken to reduce their likelihood of occurring, for example floor coverings should be safe and non-slippery; lighting needs to be adequate both in the home and institution, night lights should be suitably placed. The addition of rails on stairs, in bathrooms and lavatories may prevent falls; the use of non-slip bath mats and bath seats are helpful for the person who wishes to use a bath – a shower might be safer. Footwear for the elderly should be both supportive and non-slip; walking in slippers or in stockinged feet can be hazardous.

■ THE NEED TO FEEL WANTED, TO BELONG

The basic sense of belonging comes from relationships with others, which help to sustain life, and give it meaning. Primary relationships of face-to-face interaction are more intimate and come from relatives and partners, close friends, children and grandchildren. These relationships provide a strong sense of sharing and belonging. Secondary relationships are less personal coming from neighbours, workmates, friends and associates and are more superficial.

As the older person ages it is likely that friends and relatives of the same generation may die first; thus, friendship and a relationship built up over the years is lost and the older person can become lonely. Not all older people will be lonely; many have the ability to make new friends, to continue interests and pastimes that provide fulfilment. Some older people have pets – a dog, cat or caged bird, and they become the older person's friend and companion. If he is admitted to hospital, leaving the pet behind can cause more anxiety than the reason for admission and the nurse must be aware of this and reassure the person of the animal's welfare.

■ Loneliness

It is important to distinguish between 'aloneness' and 'loneliness'. Older people like to be alone; this gives time for reflection of the past and time for private thoughts. Loneliness can mean isolation even if there are people about; some elderly people in hospital and residential care complain of loneliness, but they are not alone.

There are many reasons for loneliness. It may be caused by bereavement as a result of death of a partner; a geographical reason is through lack of transport in rural areas, and there can be isolation in an inner city, when older people are frightened of going out due to high crime rates. Difficulties with walking or incontinence can further socially isolate a person in his own home and reduce social contacts. Similarly, inability to communicate as a result of paralysis from a stroke, or deafness can isolate the elderly.

■ THE NEED FOR LOVE AND SEXUAL WELL-BEING

The World Health Organization defines sexual health as 'The integration of somatic, emotional, intellectual and social aspects of sexual being, in ways that are positively enriching and that enhance personality, communication and love.'

Sexuality exists throughout life in one form or another: older people need to express sexual feelings particularly to their loved ones; many young older people continue to enjoy the sexual act of making love. As age increases love and warmth of sharing and touching between people may be sufficient. To know someone cares is important for men and women. The expression of masculinity or femininity should be encouraged, for older people to care for their skin and hair and to dress appropriately. These things all help to enhance personal self-esteem: if a person knows that he looks good, he usually feels good.

■ NEED FOR SELF-ESTEEM

Self-esteem is a feeling of having some worth or value, being useful and competent. A person with a disabling condition can still be able to feel that he is an important and valued member of a group or a family. By old age many people have built up self-esteem based on past experiences in the workplace or in the home bringing up a family of children. It is therefore important to let them continue to make decisions for themselves, to have a voice in their care, and to respect their individuality as people.

■ SELF-ACTUALIZATION

This is the highest level of human functions as defined by Maslow who suggested that to reach self-actualization one needed age, maturity and wisdom. Not everyone reaches his personal goal in life; self-actualization is associated with life satisfaction, a measure of aspiration as compared to achievement and happiness.

When caring for an older person it is not only necessary to deal with the immediate nursing problems, but to assess all his/her needs. Time is required to get to know him, to develop trust and friendship. There is no doubt that if there is mutual trust between him and the people that care for him, then nursing him will be easier and more enjoyable for all concerned.

■ REFERENCES

Isaacs, B., Livingstone, M. and Neville, Y. (1972). *Survival of the Unfittest*, p. 78. Routledge, London.

Maslow, A. H. (1954). *Motivation and Personality*. Harper and Row, New York.

Thomas, T. M., Plymat, K. R., Blannin, J. and Meade, T. W. (1980). Prevalence of urinary incontinence. *British Medical Journal*, **281**, 1243–5.

■ SELF-EXAMINATION QUESTIONS

1 What do you mean by a holistic approach to the needs of older people? What are the areas of need to be assessed?
2 Why should incontinence be such a problem to an older person? How can nursing intervention improve continence?
3 How can a nurse improve a patient's self-esteem in a ward for the elderly?
4 How can changes in social policy improve the awareness of local communities to the plight of the elderly poor?

4 Nursing care in hospital

When an elderly person is admitted to hospital, it is essential to put both him and the relatives/friends at ease. The admission is frequently associated with his inability to care for his own physical needs of life, such as washing, dressing, moving, feeding and toileting. As a result of this the patient frequently feels apprehensive about being dependent on others.

The areas that cause most concern to the elderly and carers and frequently precipitate hospital admission are mental deterioration, immobility, or incontinence.

The elderly patient will need constant reassurance that all his needs (both physical and psychological) will be met, and that dignity and privacy will be maintained while he is in hospital. The patient's individuality can be maintained by using individualized care based on a model of nursing. A model is made up of the theories and concepts of care that reflect the philosophies, value and beliefs about nursing older people. This in turn forms the framework on which to base nursing practice. There are models of care of which two examples are:

(a) *The Activities of Living Model*: This has been developed in the UK and is based on the usual activities of daily living (Roper et al, 1983).
(b) *The Self-Care Model*: This was developed in the USA by Orem and focuses on the concept of the patient's caring for himself or with assistance from a self-care agent (Aggleton and Chalmers, 1985).

Figure 5 illustrates the stages of nursing care.

■ THE ADMISSION OF THE PATIENT TO HOSPITAL

Arranged admission: This can be as the result of an outpatient visit to hospital; or a referral from a general practitioner; or after a domiciliary visit by a geriatrician where an assessment of the older person's health problems and physical and psychological state is made in his own surroundings to determine the need for hospital care.

Emergency admission of an older person may be as a referral through the outpatient department; by a general practitioner; or direct from the

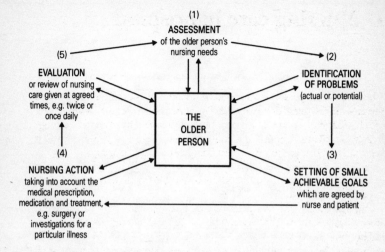

Fig. 5 The stages of individualized patient nursing care. Note the two-way response by patient as well as nurse

accident and emergency department. It may be that the patient has a life-threatening condition, e.g. stroke, heart condition, or has fallen and sustained a fracture.

■ The initial assessment

1 Immediate assessment of any life-threatening needs:
   (*a*) *Airway maintained*: suitable positioning of the patient if he is unconscious.
   (*b*) *Breathing monitored*: any difficulties reported and treated. Suitable positioning to ease breathing.
   (*c*) *Circulation*: heart rate/pulse rate monitored and blood pressure recorded; any bleeding should be controlled.

2 *Personal details* should be obtained from the patient if possible, or from accompanying relatives or friends, if any. Such details will include:
Name, age and date of birth of the patient.
Marital status of the patient.
Religion and, if relevant, whether the patient practises his faith. (Spiritual resources may help a person give meaning to his life if he has particular beliefs.)

3 *Information of family support group*: To find out the nearest relative or friend who is most important to the patient. To enquire whether there are any visiting problems, and to learn which person is to be contacted if the patient's condition deteriorates.

4 *Health background*: The following aspects should be noted:

Previous illnesses that may affect the present health status of the older person. Information regarding previous hospital admissions or illnesses.

Current health problems as they affect the patient and the family, e.g. present incapacity, degree of pain, problems about movement, etc.

The medication being taken, or has been taken, or been given in the 24 hours before admission; any allergies to medication.

A *detailed nursing history is obtained* from the patient as soon as his condition allows and any life-threatening problems have been dealt with. The nurse interviewing the patient must explain the reason for the questions she asks and explain that the information will be used to formulate a nursing care plan. Throughout the interview the nurse should aim to establish a good rapport with the patient by using her observation and listening skills.

5 *Details of the patient's personal profile*:

Observations will be made of the following and a record made of any sensory deprivation.

(a) *Visual* – Whether the patient has any visual difficulties – are spectacles worn? Is a magnifying glass used? Are eyedrops required to control glaucoma?

(b) *Hearing* – Whether the patient has any hearing difficulties – is a hearing aid worn? Does he lip read?

(c) *Speech* – Whether the patient can talk normally; whether speech is clear, slurred; are there any disorientation difficulties in understanding? Is there a language difficulty, e.g. unable to speak English?

6 *Nutritional needs*: What types/kinds of food eaten? Is there any special diet or any likes and dislikes? Are there any food allergies?

7 *Sleep patterns*: What is normal for the patient? Is it usual for the patient to sleep throughout the night? If waking occurs what is the reason, and how is this resolved, e.g. makes and drinks a cup of tea; or passes urine? Enquire what is the usual time of going to bed and waking; are naps taken during the day?

8 *Elimination*: Enquire about normal micturition and bowel habits. Are there any difficulties: frequency, incontinence, constipation?

▪ Self-caring needs

1 *Mobility*: Bearing in mind the medical condition of the patient, his age, and frailty, observations should be made to see how the patient can move about, whether it is just a case of adjusting himself in a chair or in bed, or walking unaided, or with walking aids.

2 *Hygiene*: Can the patient normally bath or shower unaided at home? Observation should be made of the patient's skin, hands, nails and feet. An assessment may be necessary to ascertain the patient's ability to manage to bath or shower.

3 *Dressing*: Whether the patient could usually dress and undress himself prior to present illness.

▪ Assessment of the patient's mental status

This can be made by the nurse during the interview by noting whether the patient gives sensible replies in response to the questioning. Notes of any abnormal response to the questioning, disorientation, confusion or strange mood or depression should be reported. Some units for the elderly use special questionnaires to test short- and long-term memory, to establish an elderly person's mental status.

The nurse should tactfully enquire whether the patient has any particular worries regarding the hospital admission.

▪ Social assessment

Does the patient live alone or with someone? Does he/she work full or part-time? Has he any hobbies or areas of interest, sport or other activities? Has the present illness affected the chances of his continuing his work/or social interests?

It is important to ask whether the patient has any pets or animals that will need attention or feeding – this might be causing concern if there was no time to make arrangements.

Home environment: It is important to record the type of home from which the patient comes and the facilities in the house, in order to assess whether it will be suitable for his return. Often unsuitable homes can be adapted, and items such as commodes, rails and ramps up to doors can be installed to enable a person to return to an independent life.

Accommodation: What is the type of home – bungalow, cottage, house or flat? Whether it is on the ground floor, whether it is his own, rented or council property. Whether the patient comes from a residential home for the elderly, or sheltered home, or lives with family or friends.

Facilities provided in the accommodation:

○ Hot and cold water? Whether the home has heating; the type of heating, central, coal, gas, electric, etc?

○ Whether there is a telephone or alarm system?

○ Whether there are stairs, how many, can these be managed normally?

○ Cooking facilities, gas, electric, Aga.

○ Bathing facilities, bathroom upstairs/downstairs. Whether a bath or shower, rails or bath aids?

○ Whether the toilet is within easy reach, upstairs, downstairs, outside, shared or commode?

○ Is the bedroom downstairs, upstairs; is the bed high, low?

○ Is the flooring fitted carpets, lino, loose rugs?

○ Is there a garden? Is it a problem to the older person?

Information about household chores: Who normally does the shopping and cooking, cleaning and laundry? Who is able to prepare the house when the older person is discharged home?

■ REFERENCES

Aggleton, P. and Chalmers, H. (1985). Orem's self-care model. *Nursing Times*, **81**, 1, 36–9.

Roper, N., Logan, W. and Tierney, A. N. (1983). *Learning to Use the Process of Nursing*. Churchill Livingstone, Edinburgh.

■ SELF-EXAMINATION QUESTIONS

1 Explain why it is important to obtain a detailed nursing history when admitting an older patient.

2 What worries might the older person have regarding his/her admission to hospital and how could these be relieved?

3 Why is it necessary to know the details of the type of accommodation and facilities that the older person has?

4 If an older person lives alone, who could prepare the house prior to his/her discharge home from hospital? Who could buy food and prepare a meal and ensure the house is warm in winter?

5 Nursing care examples

Nursing care has to be planned for each patient, so it should be appreciated that there can be no universal care plan. Three care plans are described:

1 Cerebrovascular accident in an elderly lady.
2 Hypothermia in an 81-year-old lady.
3 A varicose ulcer and arthritis of both knees in a 68-year-old lady.

■ CEREBROVASCULAR ACCIDENT

■ History

Mrs Betty Smith is a 78-year-old widow, who collapsed while out shopping. An ambulance was called. When seen in the accident and emergency department she was found to have had a cerebrovascular accident with right hemiplegia and was transferred to the acute medical ward for the elderly.

■ On admission to the ward

Mrs Smith did not respond to her name; she was semi-conscious and the Glasgow coma scale 9; the pupils were equal, slight reaction to light; breathing noisy, pulse rate 100 beats per minute. Blood pressure was 170/98mmHg. Temperature 36°C. She was cold and clammy and found to be incontinent of urine. The primary nurse and associate nurse made Mrs Smith comfortable on her left side in bed with pillows supporting her right shoulder, arm and leg, nothing was placed in the right hand or under the sole of the foot. Mrs Smith was spoken to and reassured in case she could understand but was unable to communicate. Bed sides were placed in position to prevent her falling out of bed.

Mrs Smith's relatives were very concerned to see her so ill. The primary nurse was able to talk to her sister and daughter. Counselling was given and visiting arranged at convenient times to enable them to pop in to see her. They were both encouraged to talk to Mrs Smith to stimulate a response. Gradually Mrs Smith opened her eyes and was aware of visitors, but she was unable to speak.

3 Suggestions for a nursing care plan in order of priority

Problem	Objective/Goal	Action	Points for evaluation criteria
Not rousable – does not respond to name. Dribbling saliva from mouth	Maintain a clear airway	Nurse on alternate sides Chart when turned Talk to patient Report any response	Daily
Unable to move right side of the body due to right hemiplegia	Maintain normal movements to prevent contractures of joints and muscle wasting	Place cradle in the bed; place pillow under right shoulder, arm, leg to support all limbs in a natural position Passive movements to limbs 2-hourly	Daily
Unable to pass urine. Retention with overflow	Reduce retention of urine, aim for urine output of 2000ml daily	Explain to patient that a Foley catheter (size 12) is going to be passed Continuous drainage, measure hourly Record and monitor amount of urine Empty bag 4-hourly Wash around catheter with soap and water daily	Daily
Nutritional needs			
Unable to eat or drink	Adequate hydration 2500ml per day	Intravenous (IV) therapy according to medical prescription. Record fluids given	Daily
	Mouth clean and moist	Clean mouth, 4-hourly. Petroleum jelly to lips	
Hygiene needs			
Unable to wash or care for hygiene needs	Clean and comfortable healthy intact skin	Keep skin clean and dry; daily bed bath. Baby lotion on feet and hands	Daily
		Use pressure sore risk assessment scale by Waterlow. Record daily	Weekly

Problem	Objective/goal	Action	Points for evaluation criteria
Potential problems			
At risk from further cerebral lesions	Observe any change in patient's condition	Record B/P 4-hourly, report significant changes. Record TPR 4-hourly	Daily
Unable to speak Aphasia	Patient to communicate needs to nursing staff	Get patient to nod head in response to questions. Point with left hand to objects. Encourage to use bell. Speech therapist to visit	Daily

Mrs Smith gradually became more responsive and aware of her surroundings. The IV therapy was removed after 3 days. Sips of water were tolerated by mouth, followed by 2-hourly nourishing drinks. After 24 hours a light diet was able to be taken.

A programme of rehabilitation commencing with graduated mobilization and exercises began after one week.

■ HYPOTHERMIA

■ History

Miss Lucy Bowthorpe, aged 81, lived alone in her terraced house. She was found lying in her kitchen by her home help, disorientated and confused. She was admitted to hospital with hypothermia. When Miss Bowthorpe was admitted, her Glasgow coma scale measured 12 and her rectal temperature 33°C. The primary nurse planned the nursing care as follows:

Problem	Objective/goal	Action	Points for evaluation criteria
Unable to maintain body temperature due to hypothermia	Raise body temperature by 0.5°C hourly to 36°C	Nurse in quiet side ward away from draughts at a temperature of 26°C Wrap in heat-retaining metallized blanket (space blanket)	Twice daily

Problem	Objective/goal	Action	Points for evaluation criteria
		Record rectal temperature hourly using an electric thermometer; once temperature reaches 36°C record 4-hourly. Remove metallized blanket	Twice daily
Unable to maintain a safe environment due to confusion and drowsiness	Ensure patient is safe while anxious and confused	Bed sides to be used at all times. Reassure patient Talk quietly	Constant
Potential problem, inhalation of vomit	Nausea will decrease	Nurse on alternate sides, change position 2-hourly Sips of water to be given when thoroughly awake. If this is tolerated warm drinks may be given; record all drinks given	Twice daily

The patient's general condition is carefully monitored. Any substantial rise in temperature, pulse, respiration rate, may indicate an infection, which could be chest. Because Miss Bowthorpe is old and frail and may not be able to move herself adequately for some hours she could be at risk from developing pressure sores. However, with careful nursing and the prevention of problems developing she should be well enough to return home, under the care of the primary care team.

How hypothermia occurs in the elderly

Body temperature	Room temperature
37°C	24°C
Normal	Comfortable room temperature
36°C	21°C
Mild hypothermia Shivering can occur; wrap in a warm blanket and take to	Cool
35°C a warm room	18°C

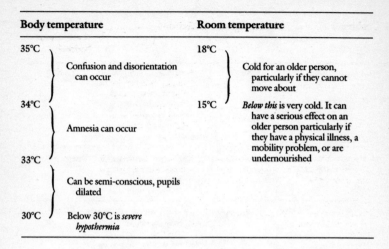

Body temperature	Room temperature
35°C	18°C
Confusion and disorientation can occur	Cold for an older person, particularly if they cannot move about
34°C	15°C
Amnesia can occur	*Below this* is very cold. It can have a serious effect on an older person particularly if they have a physical illness, a mobility problem, or are undernourished
33°C	
Can be semi-conscious, pupils dilated	
30°C	
Below 30°C is *severe hypothermia*	

This can be dangerous to life particularly if there is an underlying medical problem. The lower the temperature the less chance of survival. There is a danger of cardiac arrhythmias, loss of consciousness, muscle rigidity, tendon reflex absent. If untreated, coma and death ensue.

Hypothermia is a treatable condition and all efforts should be made to prevent it from occurring.

■ VARICOSE ULCER AND ARTHRITIS OF BOTH KNEES

■ History

Mrs Jane Brown, aged 68, was admitted as a planned admission. She has had a medical history of a large varicose ulcer, on the right leg, which had failed to heal at home with nursing care from the community nurse. Mrs Brown lives alone in a second-floor flat; she has found the stairs a problem as she has arthritis in both knees. Mrs Brown is 19kg overweight and gets about using two sticks.

On admission to the ward Mrs Brown was made comfortable in a chair by her bed, with the right leg raised on a stool. A full nursing and social history was obtained by the primary nurse who planned the nursing care in order of priority as follows:

Problem	Objective/goal	Action	Points for evaluation criteria
Painful swollen leg due to the varicose ulcer	Pain-free	Ask patient if she has pain? Give medication as prescribed; record effectiveness	Daily
	Reduce swelling of leg	Measure size of leg and record daily; raise leg on a footstool when out of bed	Weekly
	To improve blood supply to leg	Encourage active leg movements, toes, feet and ankles	After 3 days
		Clean ulcer with normal saline; apply prescribed medication and a crêpe bandage from base of the toes to the knee	

Mobility

Cannot walk due to arthritis in knees	Patient will be able to walk more easily	Physiotherapist to give exercises and treatment to both knees	Weekly
Danger of losing balance and falling	Mrs Brown will maintain her balance and mobilize safely	Ensure Mrs Brown uses 2 sticks or a frame when she walks	Daily

Hygiene

Unable to get into bath on her own	Will have a bath assisted by a nurse	Use Ambu lift to get in and out of the bath	Daily

Diet

19kg-overweight as a result of an unbalanced diet and fluid retention	Weight reduction of 1–2kg per week	To have a 1000 calorie diet. Weigh weekly and record	Weekly
	Shows knowledge and understanding of a balanced diet	Explain what makes up a balanced diet Encourage not to eat between meals	

To prevent Mrs Brown's ulcer from recurring ensure that there will be continuity of care at home when she is discharged. It may be necessary to assess Mrs Brown's home to see whether extra rails or other adaptations should be made to the flat to assist mobility. In order to relieve Mrs

Brown's loneliness and to encourage more social interaction, arrangements could be made for her to attend a luncheon club twice a week or a day centre.

■ SELF-EXAMINATION QUESTIONS

■ Cerebrovascular accident (pages 33–5)

1 Plan the care for the rehabilitation of Mrs Smith.
2 What role would the occupational therapist have in the rehabilitation of Mrs Smith?
3 What aids might be needed to help Mrs Smith feed herself?
4 When would Mrs Smith's Foley catheter be removed and a re-training programme started?
5 What advice and information might be given to Mrs Smith's relatives regarding her possible discharge home?
6 What community support could be provided for Mrs Smith and her family if she returned home?

■ Hypothermia (pages 35–7)

1 Discuss what is meant by hypothermia.
2 Explore the reason why this condition occurs in the elderly.
3 Which community services should be involved in preventing this condition from occurring?
4 What could be done to ensure that Miss Bowthorpe does not develop hypothermia again?

■ Varicose ulcer and arthritis of both knees (pages 37–9)

1 What dietary advice would you give to Mrs Brown prior to her discharge home?
2 What arrangements would be made prior to Mrs Brown's discharge home?
3 How could the occupational therapist assist Mrs Brown?

6 Discharge into the community

Preparations for the patient's discharge start when he is admitted. Information is obtained during the admission interview about how the patient has managed at home prior to coming to hospital. Records are kept of any difficulties that have been experienced by the patient. Details of the accommodation are recorded: it is necessary to know if he lives in a house, flat, bungalow or mobile home; whether the property belongs to him, or to a private owner, or council and whether he shares the accommodation with others. Ownership of the home is important particularly if permanent adaptations are made to the property, such as hoists, lifts or ramps; unless the house is owned by the patient permission has to be obtained from the landlord to alter the property, and this takes time.

In considering whether the older person can manage his/her own self-caring needs, information is required regarding the position of the bathroom, the toilet, and whether these have to be reached by the stairs. This may be a deciding factor as to whether the older person can return home. The type of heating and whether coal is the only heating material and has to be fetched from an outside shed to feed the fires also need to be established. Information is needed regarding the availability of support from family, friends and neighbours and the ability of the carer to cope with the older person, as many are old themselves. Consideration has to be given to shopping and the cooking arrangements at home, as well as the closeness of the chemist for medication, general practitioner's surgery or health centre, the post office for pensions and public transport.

The needs of the elderly patient are many and varied; functional, medical and nursing, social, environmental and financial. Prior to discharge a multidisciplinary team (Fig. 6) meet to discuss the best way of pooling their knowledge and resources to provide the maximum help for the older person. The individual cannot be kept in hospital or care if he wishes to return home whatever the home conditions may be; it is his right to do so unless considered to be actually 'at risk'.

The multidisciplinary team meets regularly, usually weekly, in the ward to discuss each patient in order to co-ordinate care. This is all recorded in the patient's notes and the care plan. As soon as the patient's medical condition improves, plans are made to prepare the patient for discharge. For many patients, going home is no problem: they are sufficiently recovered from their illness to return to an active life, with support and

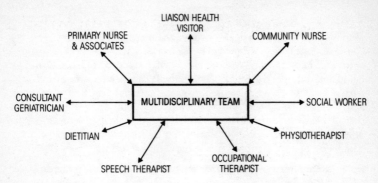

Fig. 6 The multidisciplinary team involved with discharge into the
community

help from family and friends. Some patients are not so fortunate; they may
have had a more serious medical condition, such as a stroke, that has left
them with some degree of paralysis, and communication problems. In
these cases the following people will have helped to prepare the patient for
life at home:

The physiotherapist has taught the patient to move about on his own. The
occupational therapist has re-taught the older person to dress and feed
himself, encouraging muscle co-ordination.

The nursing staff have continued to encourage the patient to walk and to
try and achieve independence and self-care, such as going to the toilet in
time to restore continence.

The dietitian has taught the older person simple menu planning.

The occupational therapist has helped the patient to prepare and cook simple
meals in the occupational therapy kitchen using such things as non-slip
mats under plates to prevent their slipping on to the floor and adaptations
to the cooker to enable it to be used without any hazards.

The social worker might have had to sort out the patient's pension, and
sometimes rent arrears and any benefit he may be able to claim.

After a period of time the patient regains his health, confidence and ability
to lead an independent life; even if walking is only possible with a walking
frame and feeding is achieved with a fork and spoon; plans can be made for
the patient's discharge.

A home assessment is made prior to discharge. The occupational therapist and the liaison health visitor (and when possible the community nurse) arrange to take the patient home to assess whether he can manage to cope once he is in his own home. They will be able to see whether he can get in and out of bed alone, can get to the lavatory or bathroom and cope with stairs if they have to be used. Any adaptations to the house are noted and arrangements made to instal ramps, rails and fittings prior to the patient's leaving hospital. If it is anticipated that the patient may need a home help then the home-help organizer can meet the patient, the nurse and the occupational therapist at home at the same time.

Before the patient is discharged home: Instruction is given regarding the taking of any medication. The nurse should check that the patient understands when (and why) to take medication, and, if at all possible, the patient should take his own drugs according to the agreed hospital self-medication policy. Where relevant, exercises should be practised by the patient and any instructions regarding lifestyle, particularly dietary changes, should be carefully explained.

Arrangements should be made to ensure that the house is ready for the patient's return and that there is sufficient food for a few days. Usually there are relatives or friends to do this, but if the patient lives alone alternative arrangements may need to be made. In Norwich Health District there is a Home from Hospital scheme: an organizer arranges for a trained Red Cross volunteer to do any shopping for the returning patient, ensures that the house is warm and that the bed is aired. In other areas these matters may be the function of the home help service.

Once the patient is discharged from hospital the primary health care team becomes responsible for his well-being.

■ PROMOTING INDEPENDENCE

Older people value their independence and the majority of them want to live in their own homes. In order to achieve this, practical help may need to be provided by the primary care team, social services and voluntary services, and this can make all the difference to the person's being able to manage or not (Fig. 7). Such help may be direct to the person, or it may be necessary to give the help to the carers so that they can have a break to enable them to continue caring.

The primary care team has to balance any risks that the elderly may take when they manage at home. If elderly people wish to live at home in their own familiar surroundings near friends and neighbours, it is their right to do so.

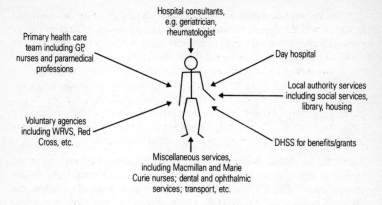

Fig. 7 Summary of support services which could be available for elderly people in their own homes

■ SELF-EXAMINATION QUESTIONS

1 Mrs Ada Brown, aged 88, has been a patient in the elderly ward for two weeks, having been treated for hypothermia following a fall at home. She lives alone in a terraced house. Mrs Brown has made a good recovery, and is able to dress and wash herself and manages to walk with two sticks. What arrangements might be made prior to her discharge? Do you think she ought to return home?

2 Mrs Lily Smith, aged 79, has been treated for left lobar pneumonia following an attack of influenza. She has difficulty in walking due to arthritis in both knees. Her husband is in reasonable health and is anxious she comes home to their bungalow. What arrangements should be made prior to her discharge?

3 What voluntary organizations do you know in your area that can help older people?

4 What can a home help do for older people?

5 Who makes up the primary care team? What does each member do?

7 The older person with mental illness

Mental deterioration does not automatically occur when a person is old. Most healthy people remain alert and capable of managing their own affairs until they die. It can be worrying to older people as well as to the family, friends and neighbours if they start to behave in a strange or disturbed manner. This may exhibit itself as a loss of short-term memory when they don't remember what they have just done or what time of day or night it is. Disorientation of time can occur when they do not know where or who they are and they are unable to care for themselves; frequently a person is restless, and plucks at the clothes. Wandering is a great worry to others, particularly if the person does not know who he is and where he lives. The older person may misinterpret what others say – often these are only illusions. They may become apathetic and aggressive. If an older person has had a history of mental illness with continued treatment throughout the years, then this can be further aggravated by the physiological effects of growing old.

Whenever possible a history is carried out in the patient's own home to observe the patient in his own familiar surroundings. The community psychiatric nurse and the doctor can take into account the patient's physical, mental, social and environmental needs and shortcomings. Figure 8 illustrates some of the services available to care for the mentally ill older person.

■ ASSESSMENT

A careful assessment has to be made to exclude a physical reason for the abnormal behaviour, and it should be based on an accurate history of the onset of the illness. This may be taken from not only the patient, but also from relatives, neighbours, home help, or whoever has had contact with, and knows, the patient. It is important to determine how long the older person has been showing disturbed behaviour. This is the 'key factor' in determining whether it is an acute episode and therefore could be due to a physical reason.

Acute organic states or acute brain failure are frequently related to a toxic state due to illness such as pneumonia or renal failure. Severe metabolic disorders, malnutrition, or electrolyte disturbance can all affect

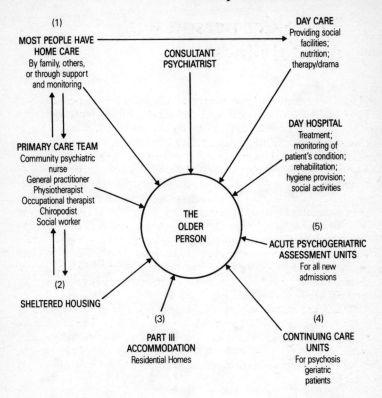

Fig. 8 Services and care available for the mentally ill older person

the brain function, as well as severe constipation and urinary tract infections. Once these conditions have been diagnosed and treated the person can return to normal. Other conditions like anaemia, cardiac failure, profound physical exhaustion and hypothermia may be a cause.

Drugs are not excreted as effectively when a person is old, particularly the antidepressant drugs, digoxin, analgesics and hypnotics, so older people may need less than the normal dosage. But all drugs and alcohol should be suspected. Over-medication with tranquillizers may manifest itself by anxious agitated behaviour. Postural hypotension occurs with phenothiazines or night sedation. A knowledge of any drug being taken by the patient is essential.

Figure 9 illustrates the chain of events that could occur if an older person is a persistent heavy drinker.

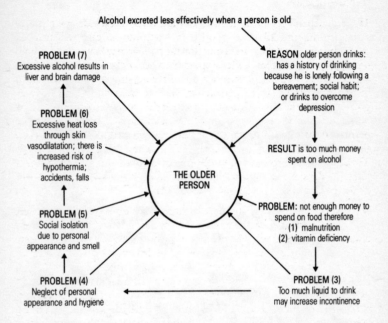

Alcohol excreted less effectively when a person is old

PROBLEM (7)
Excessive alcohol results in liver and brain damage

PROBLEM (6)
Excessive heat loss through skin vasodilatation; there is increased risk of hypothermia; accidents, falls

PROBLEM (5)
Social isolation due to personal appearance and smell

PROBLEM (4)
Neglect of personal appearance and hygiene

THE OLDER PERSON

REASON older person drinks: has a history of drinking because he is lonely following a bereavement; social habit; or drinks to overcome depression

RESULT is too much money spent on alcohol

PROBLEM: not enough money to spend on food therefore
(1) malnutrition
(2) vitamin deficiency

PROBLEM (3)
Too much liquid to drink may increase incontinence

Fig. 9 Problems caused by alcohol intake in the older person

With the help of the psychogeriatric team a constructive assessment which identifies the problems can be determined. A suitable plan of care aimed at reducing symptoms and providing treatment can then be drawn up; adequate and regular evaluation of it will be necessary.

■ CHRONIC ORGANIC STATES OR CHRONIC BRAIN-FAILED PATIENTS

In patients with these conditions symptoms may develop gradually over a period with gradual progression leading to irreversible deterioration of the mental faculties. Examples of conditions that may lead to chronic brain failure: (1) Huntington's chorea, Alzheimer's disease; (2) Other causes, including arteriosclerotic changes and syphilis; and (3) certain conditions such as multiple sclerosis and alcoholism that may precipitate brain failure.

■ Nursing care

This will depend on the assessment of the patient to exclude any physical causes of the condition. A good team approach to care will help to maximize any remaining brain function the patient may have and thus help him to live as normal a life as possible within the limitations of his condition. It requires an enormous amount of nursing skill and patience to care for a disturbed elderly person with chronic brain failure, and it causes great strain on the family and other carers if the older person is cared for at home. It is one of the reasons for respite care in a psychogeriatric unit, or permanent care when managing at home becomes impossible and continuing care is necessary. Isaacs et al (1972) quotes: 'a husband living with his demented wife found that his lifelong companion was a companion no longer; "She sits all day muttering to herself, folding and unfolding a dish cloth, looking at me, not knowing who I am".'

Nursing Care Plan: In planning patient care the nurse requires relevant data of the patient/client, as to how the condition affects the individual's ability to meet his needs. The psychological problems that the patient may have can frequently prevent him meeting his physical needs such as hygiene, diet, dressing and mobilization. Communication needs may be met by therapies such as *reality orientation* which is aimed at stimulating awareness in the elderly of time, place and person. This is done by putting up clear signs where he lives, for example, in the bathroom, toilet, dining room, bedroom, with appropriate pictures of what these places are. Verbal reinforcement and encouragement are given to jog the older person's memory. The use of *flash cards* to show simple pictures of objects that can be recognized can reinforce memory. Primary nursing enables the older person to identify his own nurse. Newspapers to read, coding of personal possessions may help reinforce memory; so also may short group discussions using headings from the newspaper or a video, and seasonal orientation, e.g. Easter and Christmas, outings and visits.

Reminiscence Therapy: This can be used effectively with small groups of older people to look back at a person's past life through personal photographs and pictures of the time – these memories can be comforting. At the end of each session the group are reminded of the present time. This type of therapy gives them personal identity.

□ *Case study*

Mrs Mary Smith, aged 78, was admitted to the acute psychogeriatric admission ward following her referral via the police and the social worker. She had been found wandering in her nightdress and slippers at 1 am the previous morning. She said she was looking for her husband, but he had been dead 10 years. Daughter has visited and said her mother has been living alone, getting more and more confused over the last two years.

On admission: Mrs Smith was found to be disturbed, confused and agitated. She was very dirty, her nails not cut and with long hair which was tangled and dirty; she was incontinent of urine. Following a medical assessment, a nursing assessment was carried out and a nursing care plan implemented. The main problems in order of priority relate to her being a danger to herself, and others, and her inability to care for herself.

When Mrs Smith is admitted she should be given constant reassurance and orientation into new surroundings; the nurse should sit down and talk to her, offering a cup of tea. In order for her to be comfortable and relaxed she may be encouraged to wash and have a change of clothes. Below are some suggestions for the priorities of care for the first 24 hours, when a further appraisal is made. It should be stressed that Mrs Smith's problems cannot be solved immediately.

4 Nursing care plan for Mrs Smith

Problem	Objective	Action	Evaluation
Communication			
Unable to talk coherently, gets cross when people do not understand what she says	Reduce anxiety and encourage to talk and wear hearing aid and dentures	Give constant reassurance Sit and talk to patient as often as possible, encourage to wear dentures, and hearing aid	Constantly
Talks about Joe her husband	Increase awareness	Explain what is happening	Constantly
Elimination			
Is worried she has been incontinent of urine prior to admission and since	Prevent her worrying about being wet; establish a pattern when incontinent	Reassure patient. Monitor the times of day and night when she is wet Chart times of incontinence Take to the toilet at the appropriate intervals according to charted times	Constantly
	Keep her dry and comfortable	Keep genital area clean and dry – and free from soreness	

Problem	Objective	Action	Evaluation
Eating and drinking			
Reluctance to eat; complains about mouth being dry	Encourage to eat	Encourage Mrs Smith to clean her dentures and put them in before eating if possible	Constantly
	Relief of dry mouth	Tempt with soft food, sit with patient and encourage her to eat. Find out what Mrs Smith likes to eat	
Feels thirsty	Rehydration, to drink 2 litres of fluid a day	Encourage Mrs Smith to drink, likes tea, give at breakfast, teatime, bedtime; water at mealtimes	Constantly
		Record amount taken	Daily

■ REFERENCE

Isaacs, B., Livingstone, M. and Neville, Y. (1972). *Survival of the Unfittest*, p. 60. Routledge, London.

■ SELF-EXAMINATION QUESTIONS

1 Following the admission of Mrs Mary Smith the priorities of nursing care were identified and a nursing care plan implemented. What other problems may she have, and how would you plan and implement the care?

2 How might reality orientation and reminiscence therapy help Mrs Smith?

3 What will make you suspect that an older person is suffering from a behavioural problem due to medication?

4 An elderly lady aged 80 is admitted with a fractured femur, and she becomes very confused and agitated. How will you deal with her? What might be the cause of her abnormal behaviour?

5 How can someone with Alzheimer's disease be cared for at home? What support can the carers be given?

8 Drugs and the elderly

It is important to remember that drugs may be absorbed more slowly in the elderly and are not eliminated as efficiently as in a younger person; as a result of this there is a danger of drug accumulation and toxicity.

Pharmacokinetics is a term which describes the processes of absorption, distribution, metabolism and excretion of drugs.

Pharmacodynamics concerns the body's response to drugs.

The rate of absorption of a drug is the time required for a medicine introduced into the body by whatever route, oral, parenteral, or rectal, to enter the general cardiovascular circulation. Drug absorption is usually a passive process. There is no proof that any reduction in the motility of the stomach and intestine due to age affects the degree of absorption, although laxatives do cause intestinal hurry.

■ DRUG DISTRIBUTION

All systemically absorbed drugs are transported by the blood supply. In the healthy young adult there are adequate amounts of plasma proteins that bind with the drug to circulate round the body. In the elderly there are less plasma proteins so that there is a danger that a greater proportion of the drugs may be free in the blood and tissues giving an increased pharmacological effect. These distribution changes may be further affected by the reduction of total body water due to ageing and the reduction of muscle, with a corresponding increase in fatty tissue. This may mean that older people have higher blood levels of water-soluble drugs and a longer duration of action of fat-soluble drugs.

■ DRUG METABOLISM

The liver is the primary site for drug metabolism. Decreased blood flow to the liver as a result of normal ageing will, therefore, slow metabolism and excretion. This will be further affected by any nutritional deficiencies, excessive alcohol consumption, or a long history of smoking or drugs. Most drugs are excreted by the kidneys although a few are excreted in the bile from the liver. Any renal or cardiac circulatory changes will affect the glomerular filtration rate; tubular secretions are slower, therefore, the renal excretion and the production of urine are reduced. This may give rise to drug accumulation and toxicity. Dehydration in the elderly can be an added problem and lead to an increased drug accumulation and toxicity. It is sometimes difficult to convince an elderly person, particularly if he/she is incontinent of urine, that it is necessary to drink more, in order to maintain kidney function.

■ Organ sensitivity

There is evidence to suggest that some organs in the body, particularly the brain, can become sensitive to certain drugs when a person is older. Brain functions can be affected by tricyclic antidepressants and hypnotic drugs which can cause confusion in the elderly.

■ DRUG INTERACTIONS

'Two or more drugs taken at the same time or in close sequence may act independently, or they may interact to increase or reduce the intended effect of one or both drugs, or may produce a new undesirable reaction' (Hess, 1981). Elderly people frequently have a multiplicity of medical and nursing problems; they may consult different doctors for each of these problems who in turn prescribe a variety of drugs. The lack of co-ordination of the prescribing of the medications can give rise to drug interactions. In order to ascertain what drugs the patient has been taking prior to admission to hospital, it is necessary for the patient to bring with him *all* the drugs being taken. To give an example of how drug interaction can occur: (1) absorption can be delayed by drugs exerting an anti-cholinergic effect; (2) several drugs given at the same time may not all be able to bind with the plasma proteins available. Interactions may block the receptor sites, preventing the drug from reaching the target cells. Interactions may also occur if two drugs are mixed prior to administration, e.g. injections.

Phenylbutazone prescribed for arthritis may increase heart failure, and steroids can bring about latent diabetes mellitus. Patients taking several drugs at the same time need regular review.

■ PATIENT COMPLIANCE

This describes a patient who complies with the instructions given regarding the taking of medication. Older people do not always understand instructions; they cannot always read the labels; they forget to take the tablets or medicines; if they forget they sometimes then take a double dose. It is important to let the pharmacist know that a child-proof bottle top should not be used. (The author has seen an older person use a tin opener to try and get into his tablet bottle.)

In order to ensure patient compliance it is important that the nurse gives clear, simple instructions and that the older person repeats what the nurse has said to ensure understanding. The same instructions may need to be given to relatives. Practice in self-medication is often a good idea to prepare the patient to cope on his own. When self-medication practice of drug administration is carried out, the locally defined hospital policy needs to be followed in order to safeguard both the patient and the nurse. The use of numbered containers to hold the morning, lunchtime and evening doses can be used; colour coding can also be used. If this is used do check that the older person is not colour blind.

If an older person's condition deteriorates this can be due to the drugs being taken; if confusion or untoward behaviour occurs it can be caused by the drugs. Digoxin, the anti-parkinsonian drugs, sedatives and hypnotics can all cause confusion in the elderly.

Hypnotics are a frequent cause of confusion at night, and may lead to a hangover effect the next day, especially long-acting benzodiazepines such as nitrazepam.

Some common symptoms in the elderly which may be caused by drugs

Drug	Symptom/side-effect
digoxin; levodopa	anorexia, nausea and vomiting
digoxin; tricyclic antidepressants; anticholinergic drugs	cardiac arrhythmias
reserpine; methyldopa	depression
antihypertensive drugs	avoid except in severe cases as side-effects from the hypotensive agents are common in old people
diuretics	salt and water deficiency and hypokalaemia
corticosteroids; thiazide diuretics	diabetes mellitus

Drug	Symptom/side-effect
steroids; phenylbutazone; stilboestrol; carbenoxolone	fluid retention
aspirin; phenylbutazone; indomethacin; steroids	gastro-intestinal bleeding

The nurse is often the first to notice whether a patient is developing any abnormal effects from the medication being taken; she must report this to the doctor. Knowledge and understanding of drugs and their effects on the elderly person by the nurse can reduce the problems of drug interaction.

Thorough and careful instruction about self-medication to patients going home is important so that they really understand, not only how often to take the medicines and tablets but why they need to take them. Careful instructions need to be given about any side-effects should they occur.

■ REFERENCE

Hess, P. (1981). *Drug Use and Abuse*, p. 80. C.V. Mosby Co, St Louis.

British National Formulary (BNF) is published six-monthly and is freely available in all hospitals, health centres and general practices. All nurses should make themselves proficient in using it to check drug side-effects, reactions, dosages, etc.

■ SELF-EXAMINATION QUESTIONS

1 What observations should you make before giving a repeat dose of a drug to an older person?
2 What side-effects can digoxin cause?
3 Agitation and restlessness are common problems in older people. How might these be treated, and what nursing care might you give?
4 How would you teach an older person who was deaf and arthritic to take his tablets before going home?
5 An older person becomes confused and disorientated; what would you do?
6 Why is it important to ask a new patient admitted to the ward whether he has been taking any medicines prior to admission?

9 Death

Death is usually a natural process, the end to living; sometimes it is unexpected and sudden – the person goes to bed and dies in his sleep; or it can follow a long illness and dependence on others. If death follows a long illness preparation may be possible both for the patient and the family and friends. The stages of approaching death may be experienced (Kubler-Ross, 1973).

■ 1st stage: Denial and isolation

This initial reaction is a defence mechanism that buffers the person against the shock. For example, 'not me it cannot be time', when told they have a terminal illness. Many people deliberately make long-term plans and deny that they have anything wrong. It is much easier if the possibility of death can be discussed with the patient and the family, and life enjoyed with loved ones as much as possible each day until the end comes.

■ 2nd stage: Anger

This can be observed when someone says, 'Why me?' 'Why not that ninety-year-old in the side room?' Inappropriate anger is often directed against the nurse or the doctor, dissatisfaction with the care or irritation for delays or treatment. People who are the prime targets are those who are caring. The dying person becomes difficult and unco-operative, aggressive and difficult to live with. This can be a reason for hospital admission.

■ 3rd stage: Bargaining

This is when the dying person wishes to extend his life so that he may be rewarded for good behaviour. Bargaining is an attempt by the patient to postpone death for good behaviour. This stage is usually short and may pass unrecognized.

■ 4th stage: Depression and grieving

When the patient realizes that death is inevitable and that denial, anger and bargaining are not effective, depression may develop. It is a time of realization that an active life is going to be lost, with the loss of family, friends and of life itself. This is a time when the nurse and the family need to offer comfort and help to the patient, for at this stage he feels ill and weaker and the thought of death depresses him.

■ 5th stage: Acceptance or resignation

This is a time of calm and sometimes a feeling of peace for the patient. He gives up the struggle and accepts what is wrong with him. He can face his family and friends calmly and will comply with his carers without being difficult.

Nurses need to be aware that these stages may not occur in order; some may be missed out, or the patient may die before reaching the so-called fifth stage. Assessment, planning and implementation of care need to be carried out in order to provide the best nursing for the individual patient and the family.

The general philosophy of nursing care for the dying patient relates to the quality of life rather than just the quantity. One should question whether it is right to resuscitate a frail elderly person who has a terminal illness, incontinence, confusion and severe deformities. If a person is dying he should be allowed to do so peacefully.

If the older person is able to be nursed at home in his own surroundings, arrangements may be possible to give as much help to the family. Dying

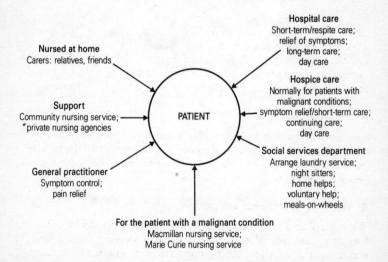

Fig. 10 Nursing care available for dying patients

can be lonely and wherever possible the patient should not be without someone near to give support and comfort. A person suffering from a lengthy terminal illness should be encouraged to live life to the fullest, with good symptom control and relief of mental and physical pain. Good nursing care needs to be given whether at home, hospital, hospice or private nursing home. Figure 10 indicates the types of nursing care available.

■ DEATH

If the relatives are present at the death it may be a help in the transition from the phase of shock to that of reality that they are aware that the person is dead and are able to share the parting. Age is not important when one has loved an older person, a marriage partner or a relative – for all of them an emotional bond is broken. Relatives may experience the similar stages of bereavement as those of the dying person, and it can take a long time before grief is overcome.

It is useful if help is available to support the remaining spouse or family and to offer practical advice regarding the arrangements necessary following a death. The funeral director is likely to be one of the surest sources of help. Figure 11 outlines some of the areas which will require action after a death.

Bereavement counselling, if necessary, may be available locally. One national organization, CRUSE (address, p. 68), has numerous local offices, addresses of which may be in the Yellow Pages telephone directory or directly from the national headquarters.

■ REFERENCE

Kubler-Ross, E. (1973). *On Death and Dying*. Tavistock Publications, London.

■ SELF-EXAMINATION QUESTIONS

1 How can a Macmillan nurse help a patient at home who is dying from a malignant condition?
2 What do you know about the Marie Curie nursing service? Who is eligible to have this service?

3 What comfort and advice would you give an elderly woman who has just heard that her husband has died in your ward?

4 How would you deal with a patient who asked if he was dying?

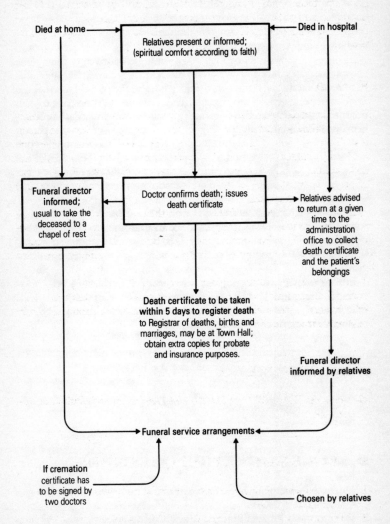

Fig. 11 What to do after a death

Answers to the self-examination questions

The self-examination questions are to be found at the end of each chapter. It is not possible, nor is it intended, to give complete answers to them. This chapter indicates the points which should be included in each answer; it is suggested that the nurse answers the question and then checks whether the important points have been covered. The select book list on page 67 will point the nurse to sources from which she can cull information to enlarge her own knowledge.

■ CHAPTER 1 (page 1)

1 People are living longer in their 80s as a result of improved environmental factors, such as better housing, clean water, sanitation, safe disposal of refuse, improved food standards and safer working conditions. Eradication of the infectious diseases by immunization, e.g. diphtheria, TB, polio. These diseases were killers at the beginning of the century. Knowledge of antibiotics and other drugs has reduced infections that have previously caused death. Improved medical, nursing and technical knowledge have treated many of the incurable conditions of the past. Improved health knowledge by the general public has led to a healthier lifestyle.

2 Yes, in some places in Britain there is a disproportionate number of old people to young people. This causes a strain on the number of doctors, nurses, social workers, home helps and others caring for the elderly. There is an increasing burden on hospitals to provide care when money and resources are short.

There is a problem in providing sufficient accommodation and care for the very old, over the 85+ age-group, and this is going to increase. The only way this problem can be overcome is to promote greater awareness by government to direct resources to where they are needed.

3 Yes, it can be a problem especially if the older person has had a bereavement.

It is important for the carer to recognize that the older person is lonely and find ways of relieving the loneliness, such as luncheon clubs, social clubs, LEA classes, day centres and voluntary visitors. Isolation can be deliberate on the part of the older person who prefers his own company. If isolation is caused as a result of an illness, or disability causing a mobility problem, then efforts should be made to get such people out of their homes on a regular basis.

■ CHAPTER 2 (page 6)

1 Psychological theories, disengagement theory, activity theory. Biological theories, waste product accumulation theory, auto-immune theory, programmed ageing theory.

2 The Norton pressure sore at-risk calculator was introduced to identify people at risk from developing pressure sores. It identifies mobility, incontinence, activity, physical condition and mental state. Each part is rated on a scale of 1–4; the maximum score of 20 could be scored by a fit patient, the minimum score of 5 would be scored if a patient was in poor mental or physical condition. This relationship of a low score and the incidence of pressure sores can be identified and indicates that extra nursing care is needed.

3 The Waterlow at-risk calculator differs in the following ways: it identifies patients' build and weight for height, skin types, continence, mobility, sex, age, appetite; and includes people at special risk, i.e. those with poor nutrition or terminal cancer. It includes any sensory deprivation, for example diabetes or paralysis; patients taking anti-inflammatory drugs or steroids, smoking 10 cigarettes or more a day. Others considered at risk are patients having had orthopaedic surgery for fractures below the waist. The higher the score the greater the risk.

4 Hypothermia is the condition in which the central body temperature drops below 35C° in an older person. Diseases such as myxoedema increase the risk. An older person cannot regulate the body temperature so effectively as a young person and there is less body fat to act as an insulator. One of the common causes is when older people live in poorly heated homes. Contributing factors are lack of nourishing calorific food; lack of money, or the inability to cook, all contribute to malnutrition. If the older person cannot move about, e.g. as the result of arthritis, stroke, or Parkinson's disease, they will not keep warm. Ensure that the older person has enough money to buy fuel and food. During cold weather check that they are well and not suffering from the cold. Use 'Good Neighbour' schemes, family and friends.

5 Ageing lung tissue loses its elasticity, the number of alveoli are reduced, the vital capacity of the lungs are reduced. If kyphosis is present it may restrict movement of the rib cage. Unless older people are fit and exercise regularly they are more at risk.

6 Adequate preparation should mean a happy retirement and should include: knowledge of financial rights and pensions, preparation for part-time work or leisure, increased responsibility in caring for health, and a healthy lifestyle.

7 Avoidance of potential hazards to make the environment as safe as possible. The prevention of falls from the bed and correct use of bed sides. Education of patients and staff in the use of walking aids, sticks, frames and crutches. Correct lifting of patients where necessary by the use of mechanical hoists. Avoid spilt liquids on floors, trailing wires and obstructions. Scalds from liquids that are too hot, including baths and showers.

■ CHAPTER 3 (page 17)

1 To look at the whole person not just part of the person. Areas that need to be assessed are: psychological needs, physiological needs, social needs, environmental needs, financial needs and spiritual needs.

2 Incontinence can isolate a person from mixing with others. Soiled clothes prevent a person from moving about easily and can cause skin irritation and pressure sores. Smell from a person who is incontinent is difficult to disguise. Soiled wet clothes cause extra laundry, wet bedding and soiled chairs, unless they have been protected. The older person frequently feels degraded and unhappy unless continence can be obtained. Nursing intervention is needed to determine a cause. Observation of the patient to find any pattern to the incontinence, time of day, etc.

If a cause has been found this is treated. If the patient cannot get to the toilet in time the provision of a commode near the bed may be the answer. It may be necessary to establish regular toilet training. Pelvic floor exercises can help to strengthen weak muscles. Suitable use of continence aids to aid mobility will give the patient peace of mind that no accident will occur.

3 It is important that patients feel that they are treated as individuals. A nurse can improve a patient's self-esteem by ensuring that whenever possible he contributes towards his own goals for nursing care. It is important that a patient feels that he has a voice in making his own decisions and in planning any follow-up or community care.

4 Emphasis on health caring by central government, increased spending on health and social services to meet the need to provide more resources for the elderly. Identify the elderly who require rehousing or finance and keep those at risk from neglect, disease or social deprivation. The

provision of advice and counselling for those in need by trained health visitors; monitor the needs of all elderly people, particularly the very old.

■ CHAPTER 4 (page 28)

1 It is important to identify all the patient's problems, either actual or potential, in order of priority before drawing up a patient care plan. The elderly patient may have a multiplicity of problems; if possible, plan the nursing goals with the patient. These will include details of the personal profile, self-caring and social needs.

2 These may be varied; it is important to find out any worries during the admission interview. The main worry might be whether the patient will get better, or whether he will manage to cope at home following his recovery.

There could be worry about a pet left behind at home. A common problem is about leaving the house unattended, particularly if the patient was an emergency admission. He may worry about the security of the house or whether the gas and water have been turned off. The appropriate authority should be informed.

3 It is very important to plan whether the accommodation is suitable for the older person, particularly if they live alone. Arrangements for alterations or adaptations take time. Part 3 accommodation may be hard to obtain.

4 Relatives, friends or neighbours could prepare the house; this needs to be planned to ensure it is done properly. If there is no one to do this the Red Cross sometimes offer a 'home from hospital scheme'. Otherwise the home help service can be of assistance.

■ CHAPTER 5 (page 33)

■ Cerebrovascular accident

1 Your nursing care plan should identify a graduated programme of rehabilitation, working with the physiotherapist and occupational therapist to reach achievable goals. The physiotherapist plays a vital role in the implementation of a progressive programme of exercises to help Mrs Smith mobilize and be self-caring. The speech therapist will teach Mrs Smith to re-learn normal speech and articulation.

2 The occupational therapist will play an important role in teaching the patient to dress and to re-educate Mrs Smith to care for her own needs.

A visit to the occupational therapy department will give Mrs Smith a chance to cook and sort out any difficulties. A home assessment will be made by the occupational therapist to arrange for any adaptations that need to be made to the home. Adaptations might include handles to water taps, gas and electric controls, rails near the bath or the toilet. A ramp may need to be fitted over a step to promote easier access.

3 A visit to the occupational therapy department would be useful to see the wide range of gadgets and equipment that are available. Mrs Smith may find it helpful to have special feeding utensils that are easier to grip, e.g. knives and forks with padded handles that are easier to hold, plates that have a ridge to prevent the food being pushed off and a non-slip mat under.

4 This would depend on Mrs Smith's general improvement and muscular control, possibly one to two weeks after having the stroke. A careful re-training programme and regular toileting and monitoring of progress are important.

5 Constant reassurance to look at the positive improvement that Mrs Smith is making since her stroke. To look at ways the relatives can help her communicate and to assist her walking and socializing. To ask if they will encourage Mrs Smith to help herself and give praise for achievement.

6 If a place in a day hospital is available, arrangements can be made for transport twice weekly. This will provide a continuity of physiotherapy, occupational therapy, speech therapy and a close monitoring of Mrs Smith's progress. The days Mrs Smith does not attend, the home help can call, together with meals-on-wheels. The nursing care assistant can help Mrs Smith to bath.

The health visitor will co-ordinate the care, monitor the progress and liaise with other members of the team.

■ Hypothermia

1 Hypothermia is the medical term for the condition of a person with a low body temperature. *Hypo-* below, *therme-* heat. Hypothermia is said to be present when the core temperature goes below 35°C.

2 Exposure to cold in the home; the elderly poor are at the most risk as are those who are ill and disabled. The bedroom temperature should be at about 24°C. Contributing factors are lack of nourishing calorific food that provides heat and warmth and lack of money to pay the fuel bills. There is a danger to the older person who falls in an unheated room, because it results in hypothermia as in Miss Bowthorpe's case.

3 The health visitor, or the community nurse, will be asked to co-ordinate

the services required. The social worker will ensure that there is sufficient fuel for heating, food, clothing and bedding. The home help will be asked to continue to call daily and to report any problems to the appropriate authorities. Meals-on-wheels could be organized to ensure that food is given regularly. Relatives could be asked to visit frequently, also friends and neighbours, to keep an eye on Miss Bowthorpe.

4 Careful monitoring by all the carers to check that Miss Bowthorpe is living in a warm home and that she can manage to cope on her own; making sure that Miss Bowthorpe understands the importance of dressing appropriately for the weather. If necessary a bed could be brought downstairs in cold weather. Alert relatives to the danger that hypothermia could occur again.

■ Varicose ulcer and arthritis of both knees

1 To continue the diet started in hospital and the advice given by the dietician. The dietician will stress the importance of avoiding all sugar, pastries, cakes, sweets, chocolate and too much fat. Regular well-balanced meals should be taken, with plenty of fibre from fresh fruit, vegetables and whole cereals. The patient should be weighed weekly and the dietician informed of any problems.

2 A letter to the patient's general practitioner to inform of her discharge home. To contact Mrs Brown's community nurse to arrange for a visit when she is discharged. To arrange for Mrs Brown to attend a luncheon club twice a week and a day centre. Arrangements to be made to contact the voluntary neighbourhood scheme to see if someone can take Mrs Brown shopping. If Mrs Brown lived in a council flat then the local housing department could be asked if she could transfer to a ground-floor flat, if one became available.

3 The occupational therapist could visit Mrs Brown's flat to carry out a home assessment prior to her discharge. The visit would be arranged to see if any adaptations can be made. The loan of an ejector-type armchair, raised toilet seat and commode.

■ CHAPTER 6 (page 40)

1 Mrs Brown can decide what she wants to do; if she feels that she can manage on her own then she should be given every assistance to do so. A home help could be arranged to assist her with the shopping, cleaning and cooking. A nursing assistant may be asked to assist Mrs Brown with

a regular bath. Meals-on-wheels could be arranged to ensure that she is getting regular food.

If Mrs Brown found that she could not manage on her own, alternative arrangements might be made with relatives. Failing this, Part 3 accommodation in a residential home for the elderly would be found.

2   Mrs Lily Smith may be given a walking frame, or elbow crutches and the use of a wheelchair. The occupational therapist will visit the home to see if a ramp is needed up to the doors of the bungalow; rails might be needed in the bathroom and toilet. Arrangements might be made for Mrs Smith to continue her physiotherapy either at home or as an outpatient.

3   You will find a list of voluntary organizations at the health centre, doctor's surgery or Citizens Advice Bureau.

4   A home help can be organized through the social services department. The home help is carefully chosen to undertake the work that the housewife would normally do, such as shopping, cooking, basic light housework. A home help may be required to bring in coal where there are open fires and also light the fires. The home help is trained to inform the appropriate people if she finds the older person ill or needing help in any way.

5   This may vary in each health district. The main members of the primary care team are the general practitioners, the community nurses and health visitors.

■ CHAPTER 7 (page 44)

1   Mrs Mary Smith might have a number of nursing problems as a result of her confusion and neglect. One of these could be constipation; this might have made her confusion worse. The nursing care should include increasing fluid intake, giving a high fibre diet and monitoring any bowel action or discomfort. If there is no bowel action, appropriate suppositories or laxatives should be given as prescribed.

2   *Reality orientation* may help her become aware of her surroundings, stimulating awareness of time, place and person. *Reminiscence therapy* may help her to look back at some of the events that have occurred in her life; through looking at photographs and letters, these memories may be comforting.

3   To compare the behaviour of a person before taking a drug and after medication. If there is any change in behaviour such as confusion, it may

be caused by the medication. Note the time of the day or night that it occurs. Sometimes confusion is worse at night following sedation.

4 This might be due to the strange unfamiliar surroundings, the shock of the accident or any analgesics that have been given. Quiet reassuring talk; avoid a further fall by ensuring that the bed sides are in position. Avoid loud noises, bright lights, or too many people talking round the bed.

5 This is a progressive disease and it can be very tiring for the carers. The community psychiatric nurse (CPN) can offer advice and regular support. Day care may be available in some areas such as day hospital, or day centres for the elderly mentally ill. This will relieve the carers for some part of each day. Respite care can usually be arranged on a regular basis to allow the carer to have a holiday.

■ CHAPTER 8 (page 50)

1 Observe any untoward behaviour in the older person. If they are sleepy or confused, if they have lost their appetite or feel sick. Drugs given for hypertension may cause hypotensive attacks such as fainting.

2 Digoxin can cause anorexia, nausea and vomiting; it can also cause cardiac arrhythmia.

3 Reassurance and comfort should be given. It might be caused by the
. patient's being uncomfortable due to a full bladder or pain. The cause should be found and treated. Instead of a sedative at night, a 'tot' of alcohol might settle an older person if he is used to taking it.

4 This is a difficult problem. Instructions should be written and spoken. The older person should repeat the instructions in order to check that they are understood. The tablets could go into labelled containers, i.e. morning, lunchtime and night doses. The bottle should *not* have a child-proof top, but an easy-to-remove cap. It may be necessary to teach another relative to put out the tablets each day in their containers, so that the older person can see them in the order they should be taken. The container should be something the older person can hold.

5 If this behaviour is unusual for the older person check whether the medication being taken is the likely cause. Report this to the doctor so that it can be changed.

6 Not only is it important to ask the patient what medication has been taken prior to admission, but also to get the patient to bring with him all the drugs being taken. Check these exactly; drug interaction or over-dose could be the cause of the medical problem.

■ CHAPTER 9 (page 54)

1 Most Macmillan nurses are based in the community, but a few work from hospital. Their role is to help patients and their families come to terms with terminal cancer and to provide palliative care. The Macmillan nurse listens to the patients and their relatives when visiting at home and can give advice regarding symptom control and bereavement counselling. Her job requires liaison with other disciplines to ensure the patients and their families are getting all the necessary help. All Macmillan nurses are RGN and those in the community hold either the district nursing or HV certificates.

2 The Marie Curie Service is only available for cancer patients who need either extra nursing care or specialized equipment, e.g. they frequently loan out liquidizers for people on a fluid diet. They provide extra nursing care depending on the needs of the patient and family – from an untrained sitter to relieve the normal carer, to the trained nurse who is able to give drugs for pain relief. The service covers both day and night.

   The service is jointly funded by the Marie Curie Foundation and the health authority who is the agent for running the service. Requests for the service come from the GP, district nurse or Macmillan nurse.

3 It is important to offer comfort and spend time with her. Spiritual comfort could be offered; informing the hospital chaplain or leader of her particular faith if she wished this. It is important that someone can take the elderly person home and ensure that she is not alone. Bereavement counselling could be offered, e.g. Cruse.

4 Suggest that this question is turned round and you ask the person how much is understood about the condition. Then base your judgement on how much is known and what the patient wishes to know. The sister, charge nurse or doctor will be more experienced in dealing with this question, and advice and guidance should be obtained from them.

Further reading

In addition to the books used as references and listed at the end of each chapter the following titles will provide a sound background for additional knowledge.

Easterbrook, J. (ed.) (1987). *Elderly Care*. (Towards holistic nursing using models series.) Hodder and Stoughton, London.

Fisk, M. J. (1986). *Independence and the Elderly*. Croom Helm, London.

Garret, G. (1983). *Health Needs of the Elderly*. (The essentials of nursing series.) Macmillan, London.

Irvine, R. E., Bagnall, M. K., Smith, B. J. and Bishop, V. A. (1986). *The Older Patient: An Introduction to Geriatric Nursing*, 4th edition. Hodder and Stoughton, London.

Shaw, M. W. (1984). *The Challenge of Ageing*. Churchill Livingstone, Edinburgh.

Wright, S. (ed.) 1988. *Nursing the Older Patient*. (Lippincott nursing series.) Harper and Row, London.

Useful organizations

Age Concern (England)
Bernard Sunley House
Pitcairn Road
Mitcham
Surrey CR4 3LL
01-640 5431

Age Concern (Scotland)
33 Castle Street
Edinburgh EH2 3DN
031-225 5000

Age Concern (Wales)
1 Cathedral Road
Cardiff CF1 9SD
0222 371821

Age Concern (Northern Ireland)
6 Lower Crescent
Belfast BT7 1WR
0232 245729

Alzheimer's Disease Society
Bank Buildings
Fulham Broadway
London SW6 1EP
01-381 3177

Association of Carers
First Floor, 21–23 New Road
Chatham
Kent ME4 4QJ
0634 813981

Association of Continence
  Advisers
Disabled Living Foundation
380–384 Harrow Road
London W9 2HU
01-289 6111

Chest Heart and Stroke
  Association
Tavistock House North
Tavistock Square
London WC1H 9JE
01-387 3012

COMBAT (Association to
  Combat Huntington's Chorea)
34a Station Road
Hinckley
Leicestershire LE10 1AP
0455 61558

CRUSE (The National
  Organization for the Widowed
  and their Children)
126 Sheen Road, Richmond
Surrey TW9 1UR
01-940 4818

Parkinson's Disease Society
36 Portland Place
London W1N 3DG
01-323 1174

Index